Separating Cells

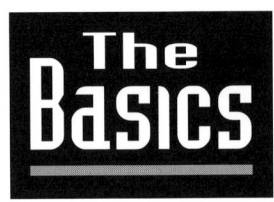

Series Advisors:

Rob Beynon UMIST, Manchester, UK
Chris Howe Department of Biochemistry, University of Cambridge, Cambridge, UK

Monoclonal Antibodies
PCR
Analyzing Chromosomes
Separating Cells

Forthcoming titles

Biological Centrifugation
Gene Mapping
Reconstructing Evolutionary Trees

Separating cells

Dipak Patel

Division of Molecular and Genetic Medicine, University of Sheffield Medical School, Royal Hallamshire Hospital, Sheffield, UK

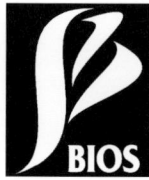

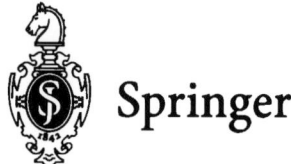

D. Patel

Division of Molecular and Genetic Medicine, University of Sheffield Medical School, Royal Hallamshire Hospital, Sheffield, UK

Published in the United States of America, its dependent territories and Canada by arrangement with BIOS Scientific Publishers Ltd, 9 Newtec Place, Magdalen Road, Oxford OX4 1RE, UK

© BIOS Scientific Publishers Limited 2001

A CIP catalogue record for this book is available from the British Library.

ISBN 0-387-91612-1 Springer-Verlag New York Berlin Heidelberg SPIN 10761145

Springer-Verlag New York Inc.
175 Fifth Avenue, New York
NY 10010–7858, USA

Production Editor: Fran Kingston
Typeset by Creative Associates, Oxford, UK
Printed by TJ International, Padstow, Cornwall, UK

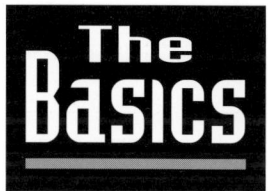

Contents

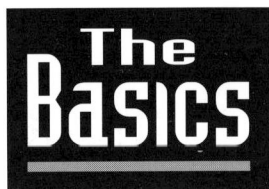

Abbreviations

BSA	bovine serum albumin
BSS	Balanced salts solution
CSFM	culture serum free medium
DMEM	Dulbecco's modified Eagle's medium
DTT	dithiothreitol
FBS	fetal bovine serum
FITC	fluorescein-5-isothiocyanate
HRP	horseradish peroxidase
ISFM	isolation serum free medium
KRB	Krebs Ringer bicarbonate
LDL	low-density lipoprotein
MEM	minimum essential medium
MES	2-(N-morpholino)ethanesulfonic acid
MS	Murashige and Skoog's medium
NBCS	new born calf serum
PAP	peroxidase–antiperoxidase
PBS	phosphate-buffered saline
SEM	scanning electron microscopy
SFM	serum free medium
TCA	trichloroacetic acid
TEM	transmission electron microscopy

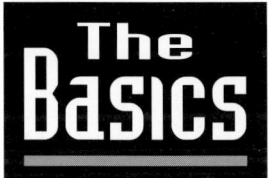

Preface

A wide range of techniques has been developed for the separation and characterization of cell subpopulations. The isolation of specific cells or fractionation of viable cell populations is an essential step in many techniques used in a wide area of biological sciences and the related disciplines. Hence, it is essential that those working in these areas are aware of what methods are available and, more importantly, which method is likely to be most useful to them. This book is directed at newcomers to cell studies as well as to experienced researchers for whom it will provide a useful update and reference text. The book begins with the preparation of cell suspensions, the first step to separating different cell subpopulations. The following chapters provide a comprehensive guide to the various methods used to separate viable cells depending on their different characteristics, such as size, density, surface charge and immunological identity. The book aims to provide enough information and guidance for the reader to decide which technique would be appropriate for their studies, to understand the power and major limitations of the techniques, and to find more information if necessary.

Dipak Patel

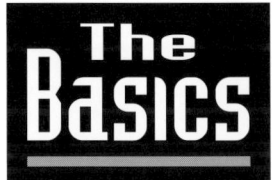

Glossary

Affinity: A measure of the strength of binding between two molecular structures, e.g. antigenic epitope and the antigen binding site of antibody. Affinity is a precisely defined parameter, the ratio of the rate constants for association and dissociation (see also **avidity**).

Affinity chromatography: A family of techniques for purification of molecules based on their specific binding to other molecules on an inert solid support. Antibodies are frequently used to purify antigens from complex mixtures by coupling the antibody to a support, passing the mixture over this support so that everything except the specific antigen flows straight through, and then releasing (eluting) the bound antigen. Technique extended to separation of cells.

Antibody: A glycoprotein released by B cells in response to a foreign compound (antigen). The antibody has the capacity for highly specific binding to the antigen. Antibodies bind to and neutralize pathogens or prepare them for uptake and destruction by phagocytes. Each antibody molecule has a unique structure that allows it to bind its specific antigen, but all antibodies have the same overall structure and are known collectively as immunoglobulins.

Antigen: A foreign substance or protein that enters the body and causes an antibody response. The name arises from their ability to generate antibodies. However, some antigens do not, by themselves, elicit antibody production; only those antigens that can induce antibody production are called immunogens. Antigens are molecules that react with antibodies.

Avidity: Avidity measures the binding strength between antibody and antigen. Avidity differs from affinity in being a measure of the actual binding strength, as opposed to the strength of binding of individual binding sites. Avidity thus depends on affinity, but also on the number of binding sites (valency) and on other factors such as co-operativity of binding sites.

Band (or zone): A discrete region containing particles sedimenting together in a density gradient.

Cell culture: Growth of cells dissociated from the parent tissue by spontaneous migration or mechanical or enzymatic dispersal.

Centrifugal elutriation: A method of fractionating delicate particles, notably cells, with minimum disruption. It requires the use of a special continuous-flow rotor (elutriation rotor), which allows one to balance sedimentation against a centripetal flow of liquid. This technique separates primarily on the basis of size.

Centrifugation: Technique involving application of a large centrifugal force for collecting or separating macromolecules, particles or cells from a suspension based on differences in mass, shape or density.

Centripetal movement: Movement towards the axis of rotation.

Electrophoretic separation: Cell separation based upon properties of the cell surface. The majority of cells carry a net surface negative charge at physiological pH. The intensity of this surface charge density varies for different cell types and allows separation of the different types by rate of migration in an electric field.

Enzyme: A biological macromolecule that acts as a catalyst. Most enzymes are proteins, but certain RNAs, called ribozymes, also have catalytic activity.

Epitope: A molecular structure, part of an antigen, that directly interacts with antibody. Typically, a protein will contain multiple epitopes; i.e. antibodies can be made to react with many different parts of the molecule.

Erythrocyte: Small biconcave blood cell that contains hemoglobin, transports O_2 and CO_2 to and from the tissues of vertebrates and (in mammals) lacks a nucleus.

Eukaryotes: Class of organisms, including all plants, animals, fungi, yeast, protozoa, and most algae, that are composed of one or more cells containing a membrane-enclosed nucleus and organelles.

Fab: Antibody fragment consisting of the entire light chain and the heavy chain V region with the first constant domain.

Fc: Originally the crystallizable fragment of immunoglobulin, Fc is the portion involved in many of the biological functions of immunoglobulin, but not in antigen binding.

Fluorescent dye: A molecule that absorbs light at one wavelength and emits it at a specific longer wavelength within the visible spectrum. Such dyes are used by themselves or linked to other molecules in fluorescent staining.

Fluorescent staining: General technique for visualizing cellular components by treating cells with a fluorescent labeled agent that binds specifically to a component of interest and then observing the cells by fluorescent microscopy. Commonly, a fluorescent dye is chemically linked to an antibody to detect a specific protein; two dyes commonly used for this purpose are fluorescein, which emits green light, and rhodamine, which emits red light. Various fluorescent dyes that bind specifically to DNA are used to detect chromosomes or specific chromosomal regions.

Hypertonic solutions: Solutions whose osmolarity is greater than the osmolarity of the cytoplasm of cells ($\approx$300 mOsm). Such a solution causes water to move out of a cell due to osmosis.

Hypotonic solutions: Solutions whose osmolarity is less than the osmolarity of the cytoplasm of cells ($\approx$300 mOsm). Such a solution causes water to move into a cell due to osmosis.

IgG: The principal immunoglobulin class in the circulation and the major antibody against protein antigens. IgG is made by cells which initially made IgM but went through a class-switching to IgG; since this class switching process occurs in the germinal center reaction, also the site of affinity maturation, IgG is usually mutated and selected for high affinity.

IgM: Class of antibody, usually the first to be produced in response to a new antigenic challenge. IgM antibodies often have not been through the process of affinity maturation and lack mutations; the low affinity of the binding site is compensated for by the high valency (IgM is a pentamer of IgG-like divalent structures, so each IgM molecule has a potential valency of 10). IgM is the principal antibody class for antigens which do not engage T cell help, i.e. nonprotein antigens.

Immunochemical staining: Staining to reveal the presence of a certain antigenic property.

Immunofluorescence: The localization of specific molecules by the binding of fluorescent antibodies to the desired molecule.

Immunoglobulin: A protein produced by lymphocytes that binds to a specific antigen, i.e., an antibody.

Isopycnic centrifugation: Sample particles sediment through a density gradient, which eventually exceeds the density of the particles to be separated such that the particles sediment only until they reach a density equal to the particle density and then band at that position.

Isotonic solutions: Solutions whose osmolarity is equal to that of the cytoplasm of cells.

Ligand: A linking (or binding) molecule.

Lymphocyte: The white blood cells produced by the lymphoid tissues (thymus and bone marrow).

Monoclonal antibodies: Antibodies produced by the progeny of a single B lymphocyte. Monoclonal antibodies are usually produced by making hybrid antibody-forming cells from fusion of myeloma cells with immune spleen cells. All molecules in a monoclonal antibody population have the same binding specificity and affinity and the same biological properties – they should all have the same amino acid sequence, because they are produced by a population of identical cells (a single clone of cells, hence monoclonal).

Monocytes: White blood cells with a bean-shaped nucleus which are precursors to macrophages.

Natural killer cells or NK cells: Non-T, non-B lymphocytes usually having granular morphology, that kill certain tumor cells. NK cells are important in innate immunity to viruses and other intracellular pathogens as well as in antibody-dependant cell cytotoxicity (ADCC).

Neutrophils: A major class of white blood cells in human peripheral blood. They have a multilobed nucleus and neutrophilic granules. Neutrophils are phagocytes and have an important role in engulfing and killing extracellular pathogens.

Passage: The transfer or subculture of cells from one culture vessel to another. Usually, but not necessarily, implies subdivision of a proliferating cell population enabling propagation of a cell line or cell strain.

Peripheral blood mononuclear cells: Lymphocytes and monocytes isolated from peripheral blood.

Polyclonal antibody: A preparation containing many different antibodies, even against the same antigen. Typically produced by immunizing an animal and isolating the immunoglobulin fraction from the serum.

Prokaryote: A simple unicellular organism lacking membrane-bound compartments within the cytoplasm.

Radioisotope: Unstable form of an atom that emits radiation as it decays. Several radioisotopes are commonly used as labels for biological molecules. Such radiolabeled molecules can be detected by autoradiography or by measurement of the radiation emitted.

Sedimentation coefficient: This is defined as the velocity of a particle per unit centrifugal field. It is usually corrected to standard conditions (20°C in water) and extrapolated to infinite dilution.

Subculture: see **passage**.

Substrate: Molecule that undergoes a change in a reaction catalyzed by an enzyme.

Tissue culture: Maintenance of fragments of tissue *in vitro*, but commonly applied as a generic term to include tissue explant culture, organ culture, and dispersed cell culture, including the culture of propagated cell lines and cell strains.

Viability: A measure of the proportion of live cells in a population.

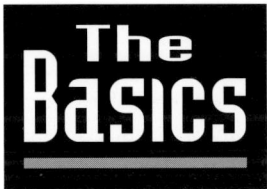

Chapter 1

Preparation of cell suspensions

1. Diversity of cells

It is thought that all organisms, and all of the cells that they are made up of are derived from one single primordial cell from several billion years ago. The cell is a functional unit within a tissue or organism and provides a basis for studies to probe the processes that comprise overall function, and/or to manipulate specific pathways for scientific and commercial gain. While many important studies have been performed on continuously growing cell lines, many other investigations can only be performed on cells from selected intact tissues, expressing particular differentiated functions. The results of these studies are used to formulate the generalizations applied to almost all cells as well as to provide the basic understanding of how a particular cell type carries out its specific functions. Cell diversity is immense and may be broadly divided into two categories: the prokaryotes (the bacteria, mycoplasma and blue–green algae) and eukaryotes (protozoa, sperm and eggs, cells which constitute tissues and organs, etc.) (*Table 1.1*). Although this book will deal largely with eukaryotic cells, it is important to recognize that much of our knowledge of eukaryotes is based on our understanding of the prokaryotes.

Table 1.1. Comparison of prokaryotic and eukaryotic organisms

	Prokaryotes	**Eukaryotes**
Organisms	Bacteria, mycoplasmas, and blue-green algae	Protists, fungi, plants, and animals
Cell size	Generally 1 to 10 μm long	Generally 10–100 μm long
DNA	Circular DNA in cytoplasm	Very long DNA containing many noncoding regions; packaged into chromosomes and bounded by nuclear envelope
RNA and protein	RNA and protein are synthesized in the same compartment	RNA synthesized and processed in the nucleus; proteins synthesized in the cytoplasm
Organelles	Few or none	Nucleus, mitochondria, endoplasmic reticulum, chloroplasts, etc.
Cell division	Binary fission	Mitosis (or meiosis)
Cellular organization	Mainly unicellular	Mainly multicellular, with differentiation of cells
Metabolism	Anaerobic or aerobic	Aerobic

2. Why separate living cells?

Each tissue and organ system is a conglomerate of various cell types. A real understanding of cellular function can be attained if one considers the cell in relation to the other cells in its environment as well as to the tissue and organ it makes up.

Many of the advances in cell and molecular biology and pathology have resulted from studies of structures and functions in specialized cells. The necessity for pure populations of specific cell types is paramount in these studies especially when biochemical properties are to be assessed and so isolating specific cells or fractionating viable cell populations becomes an essential step in the procedure.

The reasons for purifying suspended animal and plant cells are numerous. The activity itself is amply justified by the demands for pure populations as objects of biochemical research, living material for transplantation, and sources of uncontaminated bioproducts. Although histochemical studies are capable of demonstrating antigens or enzyme activities of particular cells, they show very little information about processing, molecular weight forms, inhibitors or growth factors. Any cell type with limited or no proliferative capabilities that is required in pure form must be separated by a technique that provides adequate purity, yield, relationship to cell function and adequate function after fractionation.

Cells may be separated by a number of techniques currently available using the different properties of the individual cell types. The properties used as the basis for cell separation or purification encompass cell size, density, electrical charge, light-scattering characteristics, and antigenic surface properties. These properties have enabled the isolation of fractions depleted or enriched for a specific type of cell from heterogeneous cell populations.

3. Preparation of suspensions of single cells

A suspension of single cells (individual cells in suspension as opposed to clumps of cells or solid tissue) can be obtained from either an existing suspending medium, such as peripheral blood, or from solid tissue. In most cases the cells of interest are 'units' within tissue. The cells may form three-dimensional arrangements within a particular tissue by cell–cell interactions and/or cell–matrix interactions. In animal tissue, the matrix consists of fibrous proteins and glycosaminoglycan chains in a hydrated gel, with collagen forming the most abundant extracellular protein. In higher plants, the pectins and hemicelluloses of the cell wall act in a similar fashion. Various strategies have been developed to release cells from their local environments or attachments. These are divided into three broad categories: mechanical, chemical and enzymatic.

Mechanical methods involve tissue being sliced, and pressed through filters, forced through a syringe and needle or simply pipeted repeatedly, to yield individual cells or smaller fragments from which cell outgrowth in culture is encouraged. Chemical methods are used to wash out or chelate the divalent cations (e.g. calcium) important in promoting cell–cell and cell–matrix adhesions. Finally, enzymatic methods use proteinases or glycohydrolases to digest extracellular matrix components.

In most cases, a combination of the different methods is used to obtain optimal preparation of single cell suspensions. Certain guidelines must be adhered to when preparing single cell suspensions; in particular the method used must not damage or destroy the very cells being sought for further study. One method may be satisfactory for a particular type of cell but may be detrimental to other types of cell. In the case of animal cells, mechanical methods often result in low yields of cells often damaged and of poor viability. However, the very same methods can result in excellent outgrowth in culture. Similarly, chemical methods such as chelation to break the bonds mediated by divalent cations do not produce large-scale release of animal cells from most tissue. If the desired aim were for large numbers of cells, enzymatic digestion of the matrix components is the most effective strategy. Yet the maximum yield and quality are attained when the different approaches are combined. The following sections outline methods for recovering cells from pre-existing suspensions and tissue. While the methods may be specific in some cases, they can be modified to suit other situations. The suspension of single cells should contain as little debris and as few dead cells and clumps as possible. Necessary precautions should be taken when handling blood or tissue in order to prevent the possibility of encountering harmful infections. These precautions should be adhered to when processing or analyzing the cells further either for characterization or further purification and enrichment.

3.1 Isolation of cells from suspension

Methods based on differences in density are usually employed to fractionate pre-existing suspensions, such as blood and lavages, into subpopulations. Protocols for the isolation of cells from blood are described in Chapter 2, Section 6, where they are used to describe separation of cells by sedimentation methods. This section is limited to the isolation of cells from lavages. A lavage is a flushing technique mainly of the lungs and peritoneum, which allows recovery of all cell types present. The technique is used both as a research tool, to study the various cell types harvested, and as a diagnostic tool; for example, it is known that elevated levels of white blood cells are present in certain inflammatory diseases. The cell types isolated by lavage include epithelial cells, mast cells, lymphocytes, monocytes, neutrophils and eosinophils (*Protocols 1.1* and *1.2*).

3.2 Isolation of cells from solid tissues

Animal and human tissue

Protocols 1.3 and *1.4* describe procedures for the isolation of cells based on mechanical tissue disruption followed by outgrowth into culture. *Protocols 1.5* and *1.6* describe the isolation of endothelial cells and neuronal cells, respectively; both are based on mechanical tissue disruption followed by enzymatic digestion. A similar approach is effective in several normal and malignant tissues (*Protocol 1.7*). In some cases, the approaches may not yield satisfactory dispersal of cells, as the digestive action of the enzyme is limited to the outer surface of the tissue fragments. This is especially so when isolating cells from larger tissue or organs. In such cases, digestion is enhanced by producing 'tissue swelling' during the introduction of the enzyme solution by increasing hydrostatic pressure; this is achieved by infusion rapidly from a syringe or pump. Such procedures are employed in a method for the isolation of renal proximal tubule cells (*Protocol 1.8*). Alternatively, in some cases, excellent tissue dispersal is achieved by continuous perfusion. The vascular bed of the tissue is continually perfused with enzyme solution: this ensures exposure of all intercellular spaces to the enzyme. This approach is frequently used in the isolation of hepatocytes from animal or human liver (*Protocol 1.9*).

In many cases, isolation of cells is followed by outgrowth into culture. It may be necessary to subculture the cells thereafter to obtain high yields of viable cells necessary for analyses. Since many cell types are adherent, adherence to the substratum during culture is inevitable. Cell–cell interactions or junctions may form. These interactions are often essential to growth of cells and maintenance of function and viability. When cells are ready for further subculture or required for analysis, they can be released from the substratum and each other by a routine tissue culture procedure described in *Protocol 1.10*; an important point to note when using this method is that incubation with trypsin as described should be kept to a minimum as overexposure can be detrimental to the cell.

Other tissue

Protoplasts (wall-less cells) are widely used for the study of subcellular organelles and that of genetic manipulations. *Protocol 1.11* is a method used to produce protoplasts from yeast cells. Mechanical methods are avoided as yeast protoplasts are fragile and easily damaged by shear forces. Instead, the cell wall is broken using a combination of chemical and enzymatic methods. The procedure described can be modified for other types of fungi and bacteria. In the case of plant protoplasts, mechanical methods are difficult to perform and produce low yield with poor viability. Rather, an enzymatic approach is favored (*Protocol 1.12*), where a mixture of enzymes is used to degrade the cell wall. However, this method does have a drawback; the enzymes are often contaminated with impurities that may be harmful to the protoplasts. If necessary, enzyme purification methods should be employed.

4.   Viability measurements

Once a cell is isolated from its normal environment, continued viability becomes paramount. Most viability measurements are mainly centered on direct microscopic counting facilitated by the use of various dye chemicals that give information on the integrity of the plasma membrane as a fundamental indication of cell survival. The sensitivity of detection may be enhanced by using fluorescent dyes that bind to intracellular components or by using chemicals which are enzymatically cleaved in living cells to produce fluorescent stains. Two such methods are described in *Protocols 1.13* and *1.14*. *Protocol 1.13* describes a dye exclusion method; viable cells are impermeable to various dyes such as naphthalene black, trypan blue and a number of other dyes. An alternative approach is that based on fluorescent dye uptake resulting in staining of intracellular components. Some methods combine dyes, such as acridine orange and propidium iodide, as described in *Protocol 1.14*. Acridine orange can cross the plasma membrane and stain intracellular nucleic acids, producing a green fluorescence. Propidium iodide can not traverse intact plasma membranes, but can cross membranes of damaged cells and stain intracellular nucleic acids, producing a bright red fluorescence. Propidium iodide also competitively excludes acridine orange from the nuclei of damaged cells. Thus after dual staining, it is possible to distinguish and count all intact cells and damaged cells within the field of view with viability expressed as the percentage of green fluorescent cells. Other dye combinations include ethidium bromide–acridine orange (red–green) and propidium iodide–diacetyl fluorescein (red–green); again red and green fluorescence is indicative of damaged or dead cells and intact or viable cells, respectively. This method may be used in flow cytometry (see Chapter 6).

Assays of this type are typically used to measure the proportion of viable cells following procedures such as primary disaggregation, cell separation, or freezing and thawing (as used in cell culture).

On occasions though it may be necessary to assess viability by methods that relate cell function and viability. One commonly studied aspect of cell metabolism that appears to be a sensitive index of viability, is the *de novo* synthesis of proteins. This is assayed by incorporation of radiolabeled [^{14}C] or [^{3}H] amino acids into precipitable cell proteins. Protein synthesis as a measure of viability is described in *Protocol 1.15*. However, assays of biochemical activities are on the whole restricted by the time required to identify and measure the particular biochemical event.

The assessment of cell growth is yet another measure of index of viability. The ability of a cell population to replicate itself whilst still maintaining specific functions is a good test of viability. Such measurements are used when physiological or biochemical studies are planned. The time required for such studies is dictated not only by the replication time of the particular cell type but also the time required for the selected growth assay, often extending studies by 1 or 2 days. One commonly used assay is the measurement of incorporation of radiolabeled [^{3}H]thymidine into cell DNA (*Protocol 1.16*).

5.   Separation of viable and nonviable cells

Most cell suspensions are obtained by mechanical disaggregation and enzymatic digestion, which may result in damage or cell death. Two approaches, centrifugation and adherence to substratum, are routinely used to separate viable from nonviable cells.

Centrifugation techniques are useful for separating cells that are grossly damaged. Separation is based on the altered buoyant density of nonviable cells as a result of rupture of plasma membrane and subsequent leakage of intracellular components. The separation of viable from nonviable cells by centrifugation methods is described in Chapter 2. However, although a routine and favored method, such centrifugation methods are not so successful when cells rendered nonviable by isolation methods are not accompanied by gross disruption or damage.

Adherence to substratum offers the possibility of separating cells that will adhere to tissue culture flasks. Purified cells are plated on to a flask under optimal culture conditions. The majority of viable cells will adhere to the surface by processes that include the synthesis of an extracellular matrix. Nonviable cells unable to produce a matrix do not adhere and are subsequently removed at the first medium change.

6.   Characterization of cells

The human eye is capable of discerning an object no smaller than 0.1 mm. Whilst one of the smallest cells in the human body is the red blood cell (about 0.008–0.010 mm in diameter), one of the largest human cells is the egg (about 0.12 mm in diameter). Thus it is not surprising that the development of the microscope revolutionized the science of cell biology and that structures smaller than 0.1 mm could be studied for the first time. However, light microscopy may not be powerful enough in distinguishing cells, and so other analytical techniques are used. These include:

- light microscopy;
- phase-contrast microscopy;
- electron microscopy;
- confocal microscopy;
- flow cytometry;
- magnetic beads;
- immunohistochemistry; and
- metabolic characteristics.

6.1   Light microscopy

Light microscopy is usually the first technique used to identify cell types. There are three major lenses in the compound light microscope; the condenser, the objective, and the eyepiece. The condenser gathers the light and concentrates it onto the specimen. A magnified image is produced by the objective, and the image of the objective is further magnified by the eyepiece. The size of objects resolved with the light microscope is a direct function of the wavelength of light used to illuminate the specimen. The smallest object resolved with the light microscope is half the wavelength of the light. Therefore, for blue light (wavelength of 4000 Å), the smallest resolvable object is 2000 Å or 0.2 µm. There are numerous forms of light microscopy, with bright-field being the first to be developed. Bright-field microscopy relies entirely on the absorptive properties of the cells. Cells without pigment have no light-absorbing properties and therefore are totally transparent to the condenser light. As a result, they are not clearly visible to the observer. Hence many specific stains (e.g. cytochemical stains) were developed that bind selectively to areas of the cell which subsequently become detectable when subjected to light (*Table 1.2*).

6.2   Phase-contrast microscopy

On occasions it may not be possible to distinguish the cell type using light microscopy. Phase-contrast microscopy is used in parallel with light microscopy that allows one to view the cell surface in more detail. The principle behind phase-contrast microscopy is the conversion of differences in

Table 1.2. Properties of some common dyes

Group	Dye	Absorption maxima	Type	Use
Anthraquinones	Alcian blue	380	Basic	Mucopolysaccharides
Azines	Neutral red	530	Basic	Vital stain
Diazo-	Sudan black B	600	Basic	Fat
Hematein	Hematein	445	Amphoteric	Nuclear hematoxylin dye component
Monoazo-	Janus green B	400, 610–623	Basic	Vital stain
Oxazines	Nile blue	640	Basic	Fat, sulfate, differentiates neutral fats and fatty acids
	Cresyl violet	600	Basic	Metachromatic vital stain
	Brilliant cresyl violet	630	Basic	Vital stain. Acid mucopolysaccharides
	Methylene blue	660	Basic	Nuclear and vital stain
	Toluidine blue	620	Basic	Nuclear
Thiazines	Azure A	630	Basic	Nuclear
	Azure B	650	Basic	Nuclear
Triaryl methanes	Basic fuchsin	545	Basic	Schiff's reagent
	Crystal violet	589–593	Basic	Nuclear, vital and gram stain
	Acid fuchsin	540–546	Acid	Cytoplasmic
	Aniline blue	600	Amphoteric	Cytoplasmic
	Fast green	625	Amphoteric	Cytoplasmic
Triazo-	Naphthol yellow S	420	Acid	Protein
Xanthenes	Pyronin Y	552	Basic	RNA/DNA
	Acridine orange	467–497 fluorescent	Basic	Nucleoli
	Eosin Y	515	Acid	Cytoplasmic counterstain

the optical path length through the various cell structures into visible differences in contrast that are detected as shades of gray. This is accomplished with a special kind of condenser and objective. The result is the production of an image that reveals even a transparent living cell as a complex entity with numerous subcellular inclusions.

6.3   Electron microscopy

The increased power of resolution in electron microscopy may be used to identify specific ultrastructural characteristics. The electron microscope uses electrons to illuminate the specimen. These electrons are analogous to light with an extremely short wavelength. As a result, the size of the smallest resolvable object or structure is 1–5 Å, or 1000 times smaller than that observed with the light microscope. Characterization can be carried out using either scanning (SEM) or transmission (TEM) electron microscopy. SEM allows close observation of the cell surface and nature of cell–cell interactions. TEM allows close inspection of cross-sections of a cell; it is a useful technique for accurately examining organelles or inclusions present, which may in turn aid characterization. Disadvantages of both SEM and TEM are that they are time-consuming techniques and institutions may not have ready access to such equipment nor the expertise to interpret data.

6.4   Confocal microscopy

Confocal microscopy is intended to achieve a high axial resolution. In contrast to conventional microscopy, it relies on point illumination, rather than field illumination. The system usually works in fluoresecence mode and with epillumination. The specimen is illuminated by a point source consisting of a laser beam focused on a small aperture. Time-lapse records, or real-time records made on videotape, can be made via the confocal microscope with a conventional high-resolution video camera. These systems allow the recording of events within the cell depicted by the distribution, location and changes in staining intensity of fluorescent probes. This technique can be used to localize cell organelles, such as the nucleus or Golgi apparatus. In particular, measurements can be made in three dimensions, as the excitation and detection system is capable of 'cutting' optical sections through the cell, and over very short time periods. Although a very precise and powerful technique, the drawbacks of this technique, like electron microscopy, are limited access and expertise.

6.5   Flow cytometry

Not only has flow cytometry become a very popular technique for the characterization of cells, it is also a technique used for the separation and quantitation of cells. There are both advantages and disadvantages to flow cytometry; depending on the scale of separation required the disadvantages may outweigh the advantages. Flow cytometry is described in detail in Chapter 6.

6.6   Magnetic beads

Another technique which over the years has become very popular for isolating cell types is the use of magnetic beads. The surfaces of the beads are coated with various antibodies or other ligands specific to a particular cell type. A mixed population of cells is incubated with the coated beads. The suspension is then placed in a magnetic field, whereupon the beads with the cells bound will sediment. The supernatant is discarded. The cells attached to the beads are resuspended and thereafter either plated into culture or detached by vigorous pipeting. The cell suspension can be further characterized by immunostaining. Cell separation by immunomagnetic techniques is described in detail in Chapter 5.

6.7   Immunohistochemistry

For detailed analysis of microscopic preparations it is often necessary to visualize components that are not differentially labeled by any stain or fluorochrome. In those cases, immunoglobulins (or their fractions) can specifically deliver different types of labels to a desired cellular location or target. Common antibody-mediated labels are enzymes and fluorochromes. Also immunogold is a commonly used method, whereby the label consists of small but detectable antibody-bound gold particles.

However, it is common practice to use an unlabeled primary (cellular antigen-specific) antibody and a labeled secondary antibody that reacts specifically with the first one. By this means, a larger amount of label can be attached to each antigen molecule (amplification). Furthermore, greater flexibility is achieved by the possibility of using the same labeled secondary antibody for a variety of primary antibodies. However, prior to cell staining it is necessary to consider the method of cell preparation, type of fixative to be used, choice of antibody and labeling method, mounting media, and the subsequent detection method.

Cell preparation

Cells may be prepared for immunostaining by cytocentrifuge (*Protocol 1.17*). This involves a cell suspension being concentrated or attached on to a microscope slide by centrifugal force. Alternatively, cells can be prepared by following growth of cells on either sterile glass or plastic microscope slides, coverslips or eight-chambered wells.

Fixatives

The aim of fixation procedures is to preserve a specimen in a state that resembles its natural state as closely as possible. It is necessary to choose a fixative that does not alter the epitope on the antigens or its structure. Fixation methods can be either physical or chemical. Physical methods rely on protein denaturation and consist of heat or air-drying. These are usually applied to smears and can be easily performed. Freezing (liquid N_2, CO_2, etc.) is used for specimen sectioning, and is usually followed by chemical fixation. Chemical methods are based on protein cross-linking or protein denaturation and coagulation. Examples and properties of some of these fixatives are shown in *Table 1.3*.

Antibodies

The choice of antibodies available is certainly extensive with usually more than one antibody available for each cell type. To detect bound antibody, two approaches are routinely used: firstly by labeling with fluorescent molecules (*Table 1.4*) and secondly by the use of enzymes (*Table 1.5*). Enzyme staining methods involve enzyme–substrate reactions to convert colorless chromogens into colored products. An advantage of using enzymatic staining is that counterstaining can be performed using, for example, haematoxylin. Counterstain is used to differentiate the various cell types or subcellular components. However, it can not be used with fluorescence staining as the counterstains autofluoresce.

Mounting media

It is important when mounting cells or preparations that the mounting media is compatible with the labeling media and the detection method used. Mounting media are either aqueous (e.g. glycerol) or nonaqueous (e.g. DPX); they are nonpermanent and are used in immunofluorescent staining, or permanent and used, for example, in peroxidase staining, respectively. It is advisable to limit the exposure of the cell preparation to excitation radiation and to use mounting media with an antifade component to reduce fading. Caution should be used when selecting a mounting media as some have autofluorescent properties.

Table 1.3. Properties of some common chemical fixatives

Fixative	Conc. (%)	Action	Penetration	Effect on cell components	Preservation of specimen	Autofluorescent
Acetic acid	5–30	Protein denaturation	Fast	Destroys organelles; possible destruction of enzyme activity	Swelling	No
Acetone, ethanol, methanol	70–100	Coagulants; denature proteins	Fast	Extracts lipids; destroys organelles	Shrinkage	No
Formaldehdye	3–4	Protein cross-linking	Fast, but reaction can be slow	Preserves cellular structures; possible destruction of enzyme activity; free CHO groups must be blocked to avoid interaction with subsequent NH_2-containing reagents	Good size preservation	No
Glutaraldehyde	0.25–4	Protein cross-linking	Slow	Preserves cellular structures; free CHO groups must be blocked to avoid interaction with subsequent NH_2-containing reagents	Good size preservation	Yes
Mercuric chloride	3–6	Protein coagulant	Fast	Preserves cellular structures; some effects on enzyme activity	Slight shrinkage	No

Table 1.4. Some commonly used fluorophores

Fluorochrome	Absorption max. (nm)	Emission max. (nm)
Acridine orange	480 (+DNA)	520
	440–470 (+RNA)	650
Cascade blue	375, 398	424
4',6-Diamidino-2-phenylindole hydrochloride (DAPI)	350	470
Ethidium bromide	510	595
Eosin-5-isothiocyanate	524	548
Fluorescein-5-isothiocyanate (FITC isomer I)	494	520
Hoechst 33342	340	450
Lucifer yellow CH lithium salt	428	540
Phycoerythrin-R	480–565	578
Propidium iodide	536	623
Pyronine Y	549–561 (+dsDNA)	567–574
	560–562 (+dsRNA)	565–574
	497 (+ssRNA)	563
Rhodamine 123	556	577
Rhodamine X isothiocyanate (XRITC)	578	604
Tetramethyl rhodamine isothiocyanate (TRITC)	541	572
Texas red (sulfonyl chloride derivative of sulforhodamine)	596	620

Table 1.5. Some enzyme–substrate combinations for immunohistochemistry

Enzyme	Substrate
Alkaline phosphatase	Naphthol AS BI-fast red TR
	Naphthol AS BI-fast blue BB
	Naphthol AS TR-new fuchsin-NaNO$_2$
Galactosidase	Potassium ferricyanide-potassium ferrocyanide-5-bromo-4-chloro-3-indolyl-β-D-galactose
Glucose oxidase	Nitroblue tetrazolium-β-D-glucose
Peroxidase	Diaminobenzidine-H$_2$O$_2$
	4-Chloro-1-naphthol-H$_2$O$_2$
	Tetramethylbenzidine-H$_2$O$_2$

Detection method

For immunoenzymatic staining (e.g. peroxidase) conventional light microscopy will suffice. However, for immunofluorescence staining, a microscope with epifluorescence is required. *Protocol 1.18* gives an example of immunofluorescence staining. If fluorescence microscopy is not available, the method can be modified for light microscopy by using a stain such as DAB and horseradish peroxidase (HRP; *Protocol 1.19*). Various methods have been employed to enhance the sensitivity of detection of these methods, particularly the peroxidase-linked methods. The most common of these is the peroxidase–antiperoxidase or PAP technique, where a further tier is included by reacting with a peroxidase complex containing antibody

Table 1.6. Guide to the peroxidase–antiperoxidase (PAP) method

Step	Reaction	Comments
1. Formation of PAP complex	$Ab_p + HRP \rightarrow$ $Ab_p : HRP$	HRP is added in excess so that no free Ab_p remains. If excess Ab_p were present, nonHRP-bound Ab_p would bind to Ab_b, thus reducing the sensitivity
2. Reaction of Ab_1 with specimen Ag	$Ag + Ab_1 \rightarrow$ $Ag:Ab_1$	Ag in the specimen is detected by Ab_1. At this point the specificity of the reaction is determined
3. Introduction of Ab_b	$Ag:Ab_1 + Ab_b \rightarrow$ $Ag:Ab_1:Ab_b$	Many Ab_b react with each Ab_1 molecule resulting in an amplification effect. Ab_b is added in excess such that Ab_1 is saturated. If Ab_1 is not saturated, the number of Ab_b binding sites available for binding the PAP complex will be less than optimal, thus resulting in loss of amplification
4. Reaction with PAP complex	$Ag:Ab_1:Ab_b +$ $Ab_p:HRP \rightarrow$ $Ag:Ab_1:Ab_b:Ab_p:$ HRP	The whole complex is formed and enzymatic color reaction can be performed

Ag, antigen; Ab_1, first (anti-antigen) antibody; Ab_b, bridging antibody (polyclonal); HRP, horseradish peroxidase; Ab_p, anti-HRP antibody. Ab_b must be able to recognize both Ab_1 and Ab_p.

from the same species as the primary antibody (*Table 1.6*). This is bound to the free valency of the secondary antibody. An even greater sensitivity has been obtained by using a biotin-conjugated secondary antibody with a streptavidin complex carrying peroxidase or alkaline phosphatase or gold-conjugated secondary antibody with subsequent silver amplification.

6.8   Metabolic characteristics

Another property of cells which has been exploited for characterization is the ability of particular cell types to perform specific metabolic functions which in turn relate to their normal physiological role. For example, isolated hepatocytes will synthesize albumin as a reflection of the normal role of liver in plasma protein production. Such activities may be analyzed by methods such as ELISA, radioimmunoassay or fluorescent antibody techniques. An example is shown in *Protocol 1.20*. *Table 1.7* summarizes some of the specific labeling procedures used when analyzing biochemical reactions.

Table 1.7. Examples of biochemical reactions used for specific staining

Process/component	Reaction	Demonstrates
Acid phosphatase	α-Naphthyl phosphate in the presence of fast garnet GBC at pH 5.0	The enzyme produces α-naphthol which, coupled to fast garnet GBC, yields an insoluble colored product that reveals the presence of the enzyme. Demonstrates lysosomes
Feulgen reaction for DNA	HCl hydrolysis followed by Schiff's reagent	Purines are eliminated by hydrolysis. Aldehydes are reacted by Schiff's reagent
Periodic acid-Schiff (PAS)	Periodic acid oxidation of sugars, followed by reaction with reduced basic fuchsin (Schiff's reagent)	Demonstration of polysaccharides
Succinate dehydrogenase	Reduction of nitroblue tetrazolium in the presence of succinate	Reduction yields a blue formazan deposit. Methyl green can be used as a nuclear counterstain

Further reading

Alberts, B., Bray, D., Lewis, J., Raff, M., Roberts, K. and Watson, J. D. (1994) *Molecular Biology of the Cell*, 3rd edn. Garland Publishing, New York.

Bancroft, J.D. and Stevens, A. (1977) *Theory and Practice of Histological Techniques*, 2nd edn. Churchill Livingstone, London.

Dixon, R.A. and Gonzales, R.A. (eds) (1994) *Plant Cell Culture, A Practical Approach*, 2nd edn. IRL Press at Oxford University Press, Oxford.

Pawley, B. (ed.) (1990) *Handbook of Biological Confocal Microscopy*. Plenum Press, New York.

Polak, J.M. and Van Noorden, S. (1987) *An Introduction to Immunocytochemistry: Current Techniques and Problems*. Royal Microscopical Society Microscopy Handbooks no. 11. Oxford University Press, Oxford.

Rawlins, D.J. (1992) *Light Microscopy*. BIOS Scientific Publishers, Oxford.

References

Chamley-Campbell, J., Campbell, G. and Ross, R. (1979) The smooth muscle cell in culture. *Physiol. Rev.* **59**: 1–61.

De Loecker, P., Fuller, B. and De Loecker, W. (1991) The effects of cryopreservation on protein synthesis and membrane transport in isolated rat liver mitochondria. *Cryobiology* **28**: 445–453.

Dodds, J.H. and Roberts, L.W. (eds) (1985) *Experiments in Plant Tissue Culture*, 2nd edn. Cambridge Univerity Press, Cambridge, pp. 133–147.

Kern, P., Knedler, A. and Eckel, R. (1983) Isolation and culture of microvascular endothelium from human adipose tissue. *J. Clin. Invest.* **71**: 1822–1829.

Kruse, P.F. Jr. and Patterson, M.K. Jr. (eds) (1973) *Tissue Culture: Methods and Applications*. Academic Press, New York.

Lindsay, R.M., Evison, C.J. and Winter, J. (1991) In *Cellular Neurobiology, A Practical Approach* (eds J. Chad and H. Wheal). IRL Press at Oxford University Press, Oxford, pp. 3–16.

Puzas, J. and Goodman, D. (1978) A rapid assay for cellular deoxyribonucleic acid. *Anal. Biochem.* **86**: 50–55.

Seglen, P. (1973) Preparation of rat liver cells. *Exp. Cell Res.* **82**: 391–398.

Voyta, J.C., Via, D.P., Butterfield, C.E. and Zetter, B.R. (1984) Identification and isolation of endothelial cells based on their increased uptake of acetylated-low density lipoprotein. *J. Cell Biol.* **99**: 2034–2040.

Protocol 1.1

Isolation of cells from bronchial alveolar lavage

Equipment

Bronchoscope

Bench-top centrifuge

Centrifuge tubes

Reagents

0.9% sterile saline

RPMI 1640 with L-glutamine

Penicillin/streptomycin solution: 10 000 U ml^{-1} penicillin and 10 000 µg ml^{-1} streptomycin in 0.9% saline

Protocol

1. Insert a bronchoscope using standard clinical technique.

2. Flush the lung with 60 ml saline pH 7.3 at 37°C via the bronchoscope.

3. Gently aspirate the fluid and transfer to 50-ml centrifuge tubes.

4. Flush three times in total, each time aspirating the fluid.

5. Centrifuge at 450 *g* for 7 min at room temperature.

6. Discard supernatant. Resuspend the cell pellet in 10 ml RPMI 1640 containing 100 U ml^{-1} penicillin and 100 µg ml^{-1} streptomycin.

7. Fill tubes with RPMI medium supplemented with penicillin and streptomycin.

8. Centrifuge at 450 *g* for 7 min at room temperature.

9. Discard supernatant. Resuspend the cell pellet in 5 ml RPMI medium supplemented with penicillin and streptomycin.

Protocol 1.2

Isolation of cells from peritoneal lavage

Equipment

Drain catheter

Bench-top centrifuge

Centrifuge tubes

Reagents

0.9% sterile saline

RPMI 1640 with L-glutamine

Penicillin/streptomycin solution: 10 000 U ml^{-1} penicillin and 10 000 µg ml^{-1} streptomycin in 0.9% saline

Protocol

1. Insert a drain catheter into the peritoneum using standard clinical technique.

2. Infuse a suitable volume of saline at 37°C.

3. Gently massage the abdomen.

4. Allow the fluid to exit under gravity whilst applying gentle pressure to the abdomen.

5. Transfer the fluid collected to 50-ml centrifuge tubes.

6. Centrifuge at 450 *g* for 7 min at room temperature.

7. Discard supernatant. Resuspend the cell pellet in 10 ml RPMI 1640 containing 100 U ml^{-1} penicillin and 100 µg ml^{-1} streptomycin.

8. Fill tubes with RPMI medium supplemented with penicillin and streptomycin.

9. Centrifuge at 450 *g* for 7 min at room temperature.

10. Discard supernatant. Resuspend the cell pellet in 5 ml RPMI medium supplemented with penicillin and streptomycin.

Notes

The average volumes used and recovered for the rat or guinea pig are 50–100 ml and for the human are 500–1000 ml.

The lavage fluid (saline) must not be left in the abdomen for more than 3 min or absorption will occur.

Protocol 1.3

Isolation of cells from soft tissue by mechanical disruption

Equipment

Sterile scalpels and forceps

Sieves (1 mm, 100 μm, 20 μm)

Disposable plastic syringes (2 or 5 ml)

9 cm Petri dishes

Culture flasks

Reagents

Culture medium

Protocol

1. After washing and preliminary dissection, chop tissue into pieces about 5–10 mm across.

2. Place a few pieces at a time into a stainless steel sieve of 1-mm mesh in a 9-cm Petri dish.

3. Force the tissue through the mesh into culture medium by applying gentle pressure with the piston of a disposable plastic syringe. Pipet more medium into the sieve to wash the cells through.

4. Pipet the partially disaggregated tissue from the Petri dish into a sieve of finer porosity, e.g. 100-μm mesh, and repeat step 3.

5. The suspension may be diluted and cultured at this stage or sieved further through 20-μm mesh if it is important to produce a single cell suspension.

6. Seed culture flasks at 10^6 cells ml^{-1} and 2×10^6 cells ml^{-1} by dilution of cell suspension in medium.

Notes

Only soft tissues such as spleen, embryonic liver, embryonic and adult brain, and some human and animal soft tumors respond well to this technique.

In general, the greater the dispersion of tissue, the lower the resulting viability.

Protocol 1.4

Preparation of vascular smooth muscle cells by mechanical disruption and outgrowth in culture

Equipment

Sterile scalpel and forceps

Laminar flow hood

Cell incubator with CO_2 control

Large (200 ml) sterile plastic Petri dish

Culture flasks

Reagents

Dulbecco's minimal essential medium (MEM) plus glucose and 10% fetal bovine serum (FBS)

Protocol

1. Collect a specimen of saphenous vein, immersed in sterile Dulbecco's MEM.

2. Place the vein in a Petri dish and grip the end of the vein with forceps, strip downwards with a scalpel to remove the adventitia.

3. Using scissors, open the lumen of the vein and cut into 0.5-cm lengths.

4. Take each segment, grip one corner with forceps, and scrape across the surface with a scalpel to remove the remaining connective tissue. Invert the segment and repeat to remove the endothelial layer.

5. Cut the remaining vein segments into small pieces (1–2 mm²) with the scalpel.

6. To 25-cm² tissue culture flasks, place 20–30 pieces of prepared tissue and add 2–3 ml Dulbecco's MEM plus glucose and 10% FBS. Incubate in a humidified CO_2 incubator.

7. Change the medium, observing sterile techniques, every 3–4 days. Cell outgrowth takes 2–4 weeks.

Notes

Protocol 1.4 is based on that described by Chamley-Campbell *et al.* (1979).

Necessary precautions should be taken when using human and animal tissue.

Whenever possible carry out all procedures in the laminar flow-hood.

A similar protocol can be used for vessels from animal sources.

Protocol 1.5

Preparation of endothelial cells from omental fat by mechanical disruption and enzymatic digestion

Equipment

Sterile scalpel and forceps

Bench-top centrifuge

Laminar flow-hood

Cell incubator with CO_2 control

37°C cabinet

30-ml sterile plastic pots

Mechanical bottle roller or rotary shaker

Large (200 ml) sterile plastic Petri dishes

25-cm^2 tissue culture flasks

Wide-bore 10-ml plastic pipets

Nylon mesh sieves (pore size 250 and 30 µm)

Reagents

Sterile Dulbecco's phosphate-buffered saline (PBS)

Collagenase (Type IV)

M199 medium and FBS

Sample of omental fat (30–50 g) collected in a sterile pot

Protocol

1. Wash the fat sample with PBS and trim away large blood vessels with scalpel and forceps.

2. Place the washed fat in to the large Petri dish. Mince fat to a slurry using two scalpels cross-slicing in opposite directions.

3. Add an equal volume of pre-warmed 0.1% (w/v) collagenase dissolved in M199 medium. Place in sterile 30-ml pots on a mechanical roller in a cabinet at 37°C for up to 30 min. Check every 5 min and shake vigorously. Complete digestion is achieved when the solution has turned to a yellow translucent color.

4. Add an equal volume of M199 medium containing 20% FBS to neutralize the collagenase. Filter suspension through the 250-µm mesh.

5. Allow the filtrate to stand in a sterile pot in the laminar flow-hood. A two-phase system develops over 10–20 min.

6. Remove the top layer containing adipose cells. Discard.

7. Centrifuge the remaining solution at 400 *g* for 5 min.

8. Discard supernatant. Resuspend the pellet in 1 ml of M199 medium, and pass through the 30-μm mesh. The microvascular blood vessel fragments collect on the mesh.

9. Wash the mesh filter thoroughly with 5 ml M199 medium plus 5% FBS to resuspend the vessel fragments.

10. Add 25 ml of M199 plus 5% FBS into a 30-ml sterile plastic pot. Carefully layer on the 5 ml suspension with a wide-bore pipet and leave to stand for 10 min. Discard the top 10 ml.

11. Centrifuge the remaining supernatant at 400 *g* for 5 min.

12. Discard the supernatant and resuspend vessel fragments in 5 ml M199 plus 10% FBS.

13. Transfer fragments to a 25-cm^2 sterile tissue culture flask containing culture medium and incubate in a humidified CO_2 incubator.

14. Observing sterile techniques, change the medium every 2–3 days. Endothelial cells with a typical 'cobblestone' morphology grow out from the fragments over 1 or 2 weeks.

Notes

Protocol 1.5 is based on that described by Kern *et al.* (1983).

Whenever possible carry out all procedures in a laminar flow-hood.

Protocol 1.6

Isolation of neurons from rat ganglia by mechanical disruption and enzymatic digestion (Lindsay *et al.* 1991)

Equipment

Dissecting microscope

Sterile scalpels, toothed forceps, fine-pointed scissors and watch makers forceps

Bench-top centrifuge

Laminar flow-hood

Cell incubator with CO_2 control

Sterile plastic tissue culture dishes (150 and 35 mm diameters)

Conical 15-ml plastic centrifuge tubes

Sterile glass Pasteur pipets treated with siliconization solution

Reagents

Sterile Dulbecco's PBS without Ca^{2+} and Mg^{2+}

Tissue culture medium with 10% heat-inactivated horse serum

Collagenase (Type IV)

Trypsin (2 × crystallized)

Soybean trypsin inhibitor

DNase

70% (v/v) ethanol

Protocol

1. Kill an adult rat by decapitation. Swab the dorsal surface liberally with 70% alcohol as a disinfectant.

2. Using a sterile scalpel make a single incision along the entire dorsal midline (over the vertebral column) working down from the neck end. Peel back the skin to expose the vertebral column, free the column by cutting along either side (at a distance of 5–10 mm from the column). Working down from the neck, lift the vertebral column free and place it in a large plastic tissue culture dish.

3. Grasp the vertebral column firmly with toothed forceps, and using sharp fine-pointed scissors, cut out a 3–4-mm wide strip of bone from the dorsal roof of the column. Advance the cut down from the neck until the column becomes too narrow for the scissors. Maintain this 'opening' along the center

of the column to avoid damaging the ganglia (which lie on either side of the spinal cord when looking down on the dorsal surface).

4. Without removing the spinal cord, use the fine-pointed scissors to make a single cut along the midline of the ventral (underneath) aspect of the vertebral column, effectively now dividing it into two 'halves'.

5. Using a dissecting microscope, gently displace the spinal cord from each 'half' of the column, working 1–2 cm at a time down from the neck; the dorsal root ganglia are thus exposed from their protective bony cavities and are visually identified as the pronounced bulbous swellings on each nerve trunk, slightly more translucent in appearance than the white nerve element.

6. Carefully excise ganglia by cutting the nerve trunk on either side, using scissors and watchmaker's forceps.

7. Collect the ganglia into 2 ml of medium plus 10% horse serum in a plastic Petri dish.

8. Continuing under the dissecting microscope, free ganglia of residual nerve trunk and capsular tissues.

9. Transfer the ganglia into fresh pre-warmed medium containing the collagenase in a clean 35-mm plastic Petri dish. Incubate the ganglia for 1.5 h at 37°C with collagenase solution. Thereafter, carefully remove the solution, and replace with 2–3 ml of fresh enzyme solution. Incubate for a further 1.5 h.

10. Transfer the ganglia to a sterile 15 ml plastic conical centrifuge tube, pellet the ganglia by centrifugation at 200 g for 4 min. Discard supernatant and wash pellet twice with sterile Ca^{2+}- and Mg^{2+}-free PBS.

11. Resuspend the ganglia in 2–3 ml of PBS containing 0.25% (w/v) trypsin and incubate for 30 min. Wash three times in medium plus 10% horse serum, DNase (80 μg ml^{-1}), and soybean trypsin inhibitor (100 μg ml^{-1}).

12. By repeated (six to ten times) pipetting with a siliconized Pasteur pipet produce a single cell suspension of the digested and softened ganglia. The ganglia should break up fairly readily, and a cloudy suspension of cells should appear.

Notes

A variety of media can be used, including Eagles MEM, Dulbecco's modified Eagle's medium (DMEM), Ham's F12 or F14 media.

The 'cleaning' procedure in step 8 is important because it aids enzymatic digestion and reduces the severity of the mechanical shearing required to dissociate the tissue, hence improving cell yields.

The collagenase concentration should be approximately 0.125% (w/v), but this will depend on the activity of a particular batch of the enzyme, so this should be tested in pilot experiments.

Use good quality trypsin for digestion.

DNase and soybean trypsin inhibitor may not be essential; this depends on the severity of enzymatic digestion and the quality of cells liberated, which can be evaluated in pilot experiments.

Excessive mechanical force will reduce the yield of viable neurons. Adjustments to the digestion process may be required.

The isolated cell suspension will yield a mixed culture of neuronal and nonneuronal cells; see Lindsay et al. (1991) for procedures for further enrichment.

Protocol 1.7

Disaggregation of embryonic and normal and malignant tissues

Equipment

Sterile scalpel and forceps

Petri dishes

Plastic pipets

Centrifuge tubes

Universal containers

Tissue culture flasks

Incubator

Bench-top centrifuge

Reagents

Balanced salts solution (BSS)

Culture medium

Collagenase

Protocol

1. Transfer excised tissue to a sterile petri dish containing fresh sterile BSS and rinse.

2. Transfer tissue to a second dish. Dissect off unwanted tissue such as fat or necrotic material, and chop finely with crossed scalpels to about 1 mm^3 pieces.

3. Transfer by pipet (10–20 ml with wide bore tip) to a 15- or 50-ml sterile centrifuge tube or universal container (wet the inside of the pipet first with BSS or the pieces will stick). Allow the pieces to settle.

4. Wash by resuspending the pieces in BSS, allowing the pieces to settle, and removing the supernatant fluid, two or three times.

5. Transfer 20–30 pieces to one 25-cm^2 flask and 100–200 pieces to a second flask.

6. Drain off BSS and add 4.5 ml growth medium with serum to each flask.

7. Add 0.5 ml crude collagenase, 2000 U ml^{-1}, to give a final concentration of 200 U ml^{-1} collagenase.

8. Incubate at 36.5°C for 4–48 h without agitation. Tumor tissue may be left up to 5 days or more if disaggregation is low, e.g. in scirrhous carcinomas of breast or colon.

9. Check for effective disaggregation by gently rocking the flask; the pieces of tissue will 'smear' on the bottom of the flask and, with moderate agitation, will break up into single cells and small clusters.

10. After complete disaggregation has occurred (or after supernatant cells are collected after allowing clusters to settle – see Note 2), centrifuge cells at 50–100 *g* for 30 min.

11. Discard supernatant, resuspend cells, combine pellets in 5 ml medium, and seed 25 cm² culture flask.

12. Replace medium after 48 h.

Notes

If the pH fell during collagenase treatment (to pH 6.5 or less by 48 h), dilute two- to three-fold in medium after removing the collagenase.

With some tissues, such as lung, kidney, and colon or breast carcinoma, small clusters of epithelial cells can be seen to resist the collagenase and may be separated from the rest by allowing them to settle for about 2 min. If these clusters are further washed with BSS by resuspension and settling and the sediment seeded in medium, they will form healthy islands of epithelial cells. Epithelial cells generally survive better if not completely dissociated.

Some cells, particularly macrophages, may adhere to the first flask during the collagenase incubation. Transferring the cells to a fresh flask after collagenase treatment (and removal) removes many of the macrophages from the culture. The first flask may be cultured as well if required. Light trypsinization will remove any adherent cells other than macrophages.

Protocol 1.8

Separation of renal proximal tubule cells by tissue swelling and enzymatic digestion

Equipment

Sterile scalpel and forceps

Glass beaker

Laminar flow-hood

Sterile 50-ml syringes

Polished smooth stainless steel cannula (o.d. 3 mm)

Glass Dounce homogenizer and pestle, loose bore

Nylon screening fabric (250- and 85-μm pore sizes)

Glass beakers sterilized by dry heat

Magnetic stirrer

Plastic-coated magnetic stirrer bars and stirrer plate

Bench-top centrifuge

Cell incubator with CO_2 control

Tissue culture flasks

Reagents

Barbiturates, e.g. Hypnorm

Serum free medium (SFM): for 6 l use 31.8 g powdered Ham's F12 medium, 40.1 g powdered Dulbecco's MEM, 21.5 g Hepes and 0.0072 g $NaHCO_3$, stored frozen. On the day of use, thaw and add (for 2 l) 2.2 g penicillin and 0.24 g streptomycin to form isolation medium (ISFM)

Culture medium (CSFM): to ISFM add bovine insulin (5 μg ml^{-1}), human transferrin (5 μg ml^{-1}) and hydrocortisone (5 × 10^{-8} M) on day of culture

Iron oxide for perfusion

Collagenase (Type IV) and Soybean trypsin inhibitor: add 0.05 g of each to 100 ml ISFM medium, warm to 37°C

Protocol

1. Anesthetize male albino rabbit with intravenous injection of barbiturates. Shave the abdomen and make a midline incision.

2. Excise kidneys with 1 cm of renal artery attached; administer terminal anesthetic dose.

3. Place the kidneys in a beaker of chilled ISFM and transfer to the laminar flow-hood.

4. Cannulate each renal artery with the polished cannula attached to a 50-ml syringe containing iron oxide solution. Flush through each kidney with 30 ml iron oxide solution by slow injection.

5. Wash kidneys in fresh ISFM, peel off the outer capsule with forceps, and cut the kidneys transversely into disks (0.5–1 cm thick). Dissect out the cortex.

6. With four strokes of the Dounce homogenizer, homogenize the pieces of cortex in 10 ml ISFM.

7. Sieve the homogenate, first through the 250-μm mesh, and then through the 85-μm mesh to collect the tubule fragments (on top).

8. Wash through with 50 ml ISFM. Scrape off the pellet and resuspend in 50 ml ISFM in a sterile plastic pot.

9. Use a sterile magnetic stirrer bar to collect iron-laden glomeruli. Remove gently after 2–3 min. Repeat with a second magnetic bar.

10. Add soybean trypsin inhibitor and collagenase to final concentration of 0.05 mg ml^{-1} each and incubate for 5 min at 37°C with occasional agitation of the suspension.

11. Centrifuge at 200 *g* for 5 min, discard the supernatant, add fresh ISFM, and repeat the washing step.

12. Resuspend the final pellet in 400 ml CSFM. Transfer suspension to sterile culture flasks in a humidified CO_2 incubator.

13. Observing sterile techniques, change medium after 2 days, then every 3–4 days. Primary cultures of tubule cells with 'domed' morphology develop over several days.

Notes

Iron oxide for perfusion: dissolve 2.6 g NaOH and 20 g KNO_3 in 100 ml sterile, oxygen-saturated water, and dissolve 9 g $FeSO_4$ in 100 ml sterile, oxygen-saturated water. Mix the solutions and boil for 20 min. Stand on magnetic plate to collect the precipitate, remove the supernatant, and wash with fresh sterile water. Repeat five times. Resuspend in 2 l of sterile 0.9% NaCl solution, and autoclave. On day of use, dilute 5 ml to 100 ml sterile saline.

Rabbits of 2–3 kg in weight may be sedated by intramuscular injection of 0.4 ml Hypnorm, followed after a period of 15–20 min by intravenous injection of barbiturates into an ear vein.

The cortex can be easily seen as a pale colored rim of tissue around the outside of each tissue disk.

Protocol 1.9

Preparation of rat hepatocytes by continuous perfusion with enzyme solution

Equipment

Water bath

Cylinder of oxygen gas

Sterile nylon cannula (o.d. 1.5 mm)

Sterile scalpels and forceps

Roller pump and sterile circuit made from nylon/silicone tubing

A stainless steel sieve (approximate pore size 1 mm) sterilized by autoclaving

Nylon mesh sieve (100-μm pore size)

Laminar flow-hood

Bench-top centrifuge

Sterile 30-ml plastic pots

Wide bore plastic pipets

Hemocytometer slide for cell counting

Reagents

Barbiturates, e.g. Hypnorm

Ca^{2+}- and Mg^{2+}-free Hank's BSS

Leibovitz L15 medium, 1.19 g Hepes buffer and 1 ml insulin (100 U ml^{-1}) pH to 7.4 with 1 M NaOH

Collagenase

Protocol

1. Anesthetize a rat of approximately 200–300 g body weight by inhalation anesthetic and intramuscular injection of barbiturates.

2. Warm Hank's BSS L15 medium in the water bath at 37°C. Bubble 100% oxygen gas into the medium for 15–20 min. Place the pump input tubing into the L15 medium and fill the circuit plus attached cannula.

3. Shave the abdomen, make a midline incision and insert the cannula into the portal vein of the liver.

4. Switch on the pump at a flow rate of 20–30 ml min^{-1}, and cut the vena cavae below the liver to allow outflow. Kill the animal by cardiac section.

5. Pump 150 ml L15 medium through the liver to wash out the blood.

6. Stop the pump briefly, switch the pump input tubing into the Hank's BSS solution. Pump 500 ml of warmed solution through the liver at a flow rate of 40–50 ml min^{-1}. During this time, dissolve collagenase (0.1 U ml^{-1}) in the remaining L15 medium and add to the reservoir of the recirculating system.

7. Stop the pump, remove the liver (with cannula still in place) from the carcass. Attach the cannula to the recirculating system and perfuse for up to 20 min with the collagenase solution.

8. Check the progression of digestion by pressing the liver lobes with a smooth-ended probe or glass rod. The appearance of fluid-filled indentations under the probe indicates the end-point of digestion.

9. Transfer the liver with 20–30 ml of collagenase solution into a sterile 200-ml plastic Petri dish and place in the laminar flow-hood. Gently tease apart the liver lobes using sterile scalpel and forceps.

10. Pass the slurry through the sterile stainless steel filter into a sterile plastic pot. Pipet the slurry up and down two or three times with a wide-bored plastic pipet to enhance cell separation. Divide the slurry into two 30-ml aliquots.

11. Centrifuge at 50 *g* for 3 min.

12. Discard the supernatant, replace with fresh medium, and mix with a wide-bore pipet. Repeat this washing procedure twice more resuspending the final pellet in 20 ml of L15 medium.

13. Pass this suspension through the 100-μm nylon mesh to give the final cell preparation.

14. Determine the cell yield and viability using a hemocytometer.

Notes

Protocol 1.9 is based on that described by Seglen (1973).

Roller pump and sterile circuit; the system must recirculate medium at flow rates of 40–60 ml min^{-1}, usually perfusing the liver from a hydrostatic pressure head of 30–50 cm H$_2$O.

Venous outflow should be allowed to drain freely immediately perfusion is started, otherwise poor clearance of blood may result. In practice, it is convenient to arrange outflow drain into a sink or plastic bowl to avoid flooding the bench.

Protocol 1.10

Release of cultured cells from substratum by trypsinization

Equipment

Laminar flow-hood

Bench-top centrifuge

Sterile plastic pipets

Centrifuge tubes

Reagents

Dulbecco's PBS without Ca^{2+} and Mg^{2+}

Trypsin/EDTA solution; 5 g porcine trypsin and 2 g EDTA per liter

Dulbecco's MEM plus 20% new born calf serum (NBCS)

Protocol

1. Dilute the trypsin/EDTA solution 1/10 with pre-warmed PBS minus Ca^{2+} and Mg^{2+}.

2. Remove the cell culture supernatants with a sterile pipet and wash the flasks with 3 ml of PBS without Ca^{2+} and Mg^{2+}.

3. Add 3 ml of diluted trypsin/EDTA to each flask and place in the incubator at 37°C. Check digestion every 1–2 min by gently rocking the flasks. Remove the flasks from the incubator as soon as the cells have been released into suspension.

4. Add an excess (at least two-fold) of pre-warmed MEM plus 20% NBCS to inhibit the proteolytic action.

5. Transfer the suspension to sterile centrifuge tubes.

6. Centrifuge at 400 **g** for 5 min to pellet the cells. Resuspend the pellets in fresh MEM, centrifuge, and discard the supernatant.

7. Resuspend the cells in the medium (tissue culture or isotonic buffer) of choice. Determine cell concentration using a hemocytometer. Subculture at the required concentration into fresh flasks or use for analyses.

Notes

Where possible, perform procedures in a laminar flow-hood.

The volumes are used for 25-cm² flasks.

Trypsin has a well-recognized digestive effect on cell membrane components and prolonged exposure will often prove lethal.

Protocol 1.11

Isolation of yeast protoplasts (spheroplasts)

Equipment

Bench-top centrifuge

Centrifuge tubes

Spectrophotometer

Reagents

Yeast extract

Bacto-peptone

Glucose

Tris buffer

Dithiothreitol (DTT)

Lyticase

Sorbitol

Potassium phosphate

Sucrose

Ficoll 400

2-(*N*-morpholino)ethanesulfonic acid (MES)

Protocol

1. Grow yeast cells to their early/mid logarithmic phase in growth medium containing 1% (w/v) yeast extract, 2% (w/v) Bacto-peptone, and 2–5% (w/v) glucose.

2. Centrifuge at 3000 g for 5 min at room temperature.

3. Resuspend cells in distilled water, centrifuge, and resuspend at 20 U ml^{-1} (OD$_{600}$) in 0.1 M Tris sulfate pH 9.4, 10 mm DTT for 10 min.

4. Wash the cells in 1.2 M sorbitol and resuspend to 50 U ml^{-1} (OD$_{600}$) in buffer containing 1.2 M sorbitol, 10 mm potassium phosphate pH 7.2.

5. Add Lyticase (10–25 U/OD$_{600}$ unit of cells).

6. Add 0.5% yeast extract and 1% Bacto-peptone. Incubate for 45 min with gentle shaking at 25°C, by which time protoplast formation should be completed.

7. To recover the protoplasts centrifuge at **4000 g** for 10 min at 4°C through a cushion of 0.8 M sucrose, 1.5% (w/v) Ficoll 400, 20 mm MES pH 6.5.

Notes

Step 3 is performed to loosen the outer mannoprotein layer to allow attack of the underlying $\beta(1-3)$ glucan layer by the Lyticase.

Step 6 is performed to ensure that metabolically active protoplasts are obtained.

Protocol 1.12

Isolation of plant protoplasts

Equipment

Scalpel and pointed forceps

Petri dishes

Parafilm

Aluminum foil

Nylon mesh (45-μm pore size)

Wide-bore 10-ml pipets

Wide-bore Pasteur pipets

Bench-top centrifuge with swing-out rotor

Centrifuge tubes

Reagents

Mature leaves from a suitable plant

250 ml sodium hypochlorite solution (2.5% v/v), with 2 ml of Triton X-100

Mannitol

10 ml enzyme mixture containing Macerozyme R-10 (0.5% w/v) plus cellulase Onozuka R-10 (2.0% w/v) dissolved in 13% (w/v) mannitol pH 5.4

800 ml Murashige and Skoog's medium (MS) containing 13% (w/v) mannitol pH 5.4

Protocol

1. Ensure medium and reagents are sterilized as required making sure not to denature the enzymes.

2. Rinse 1 g leaves in tap water.

3. Immerse the leaves in the hypochlorite/Triton solution for 10 min.

4. Rinse the leaves three times in MS medium containing 13% mannitol pH 5.4.

5. During the final rinse, remove the lower epidermis with pointed forceps; insert the point of the forceps at the junction of the main vein and strip the epidermal layer towards the edge of the lamina. If this fails allow the leaf to wilt and try again. If this fails then score the epidermis several times with a scalpel blade to facilitate entry of the enzyme.

6. Cut the leaves into sections and immerse the peeled leaf sections in a Petri dish containing 10 ml sterile enzyme solution.

7. Seal the Petri dish with Parafilm and wrap in aluminum foil. Leave overnight at room temperature.

8. Carefully tease the leaf strips gently to release the protoplasts.

9. Filter the enzyme solution containing the protoplasts through a 45-μm nylon mesh; this will remove debris.

10. Centrifuge the filtrate at 75 g for 5 min.

11. Aspirate the supernatant. Resuspend the pellet in 10 ml of MS culture medium containing 13% mannitol.

12. Wash three times with MS culture medium; centrifuge as before. Resuspend protoplasts gently to avoid damage.

Notes

Protocol 1.12 is based on that described by Dodds and Roberts (1985).

Two most commonly used species are the *Petunia* sp. and *Hyoscyamus niger* (henbane).

Avoid use of any fungicides or insecticides during the growth of the plants.

When developing a technique for each plant it may be necessary to experiment with various enzyme mixtures and mannitol concentrations (typically 8–15%). Lower concentrations of mannitol will cause fusion of protoplasts. It is important that the osmolality and pH are the same between solutions.

A typical yield of mesophyll protoplasts is $2–5 \times 10^6$ g^{-1} of leaf tissue.

Protocol 1.13

Cell viability determined by trypan blue exclusion

Equipment

Light microscope

Hemocytometer counting chamber and coverslip

Bench-top centrifuge

Pasteur pipets

Pipets

Reagents

Cell suspension

Dulbecco's PBS

Trypan blue dye solution

Protocol

1. Fix the coverslip with firm and even pressure on to the hemocytometer chamber.

2. Centrifuge the cell suspension (200–500 *g* depending on cell size) to concentrate cells. Discard the supernatant and resuspend the cells carefully in the chosen volume of PBS.

3. Mix 50 μl of cell suspension with 950 μl trypan blue solution.

4. Transfer a sample into the hemocytometer chamber, and under the microscope count the numbers of clear, unstained cells, and total cell numbers within the squares of the chamber.

5. Calculate viability as percentage of unstained cells in the total population. This can be related back to the original suspension knowing the volume of the chamber (usually 0.1 mm^3 per large square), the dilution factor (in this case ×20), and the volume of original suspension.

Notes

Trypan blue dye solution: add 0.4 g of trypan blue dye, 0.81 g NaCl, 0.006 g KH$_2$PO$_4$, and 0.05 g methyl hydroxybenzoate (preservative) to 95 ml double distilled water. Heat to boiling in a glass beaker and allow to cool. Adjust the pH to 7.2–7.3 with NaOH solution, and adjust the volume to 100 ml. Finally pass through a 5-μm filter.

Step 1 is achieved by breathing lightly on the chamber to deposit a thin film of moisture, and pushing down on the coverslip with each thumb on opposite sides of the chamber.

Dissolved proteins in the medium can cause a high background staining, and thus protein-free resuspension medium (e.g. PBS) is recommended; trypan blue has a great affinity for proteins (Kruse and Patterson, 1973).

Prolonged exposure to trypan blue dye (>30 min) results in progressively more cells accumulating the dye.

If large cells are under study, they may sediment if left to stand in the dye and thus errors in counting will follow.

Protocol 1.14

Cell viability determined by fluorescence staining methods

Equipment

Fluorescent microscope with FITC filter set at excitation 490 nm, emission 510 nm

Bench-top centrifuge

Microscope slides

Pipets

Pasteur pipets

Microcentrifuge tubes

Reagents

PBS

Acridine orange and propidium iodide dyes, dissolved in PBS

Protocol

1. Centrifuge the cell suspension (at 200–500 **g**).

2. Discard the supernatant, and resuspend the pelleted cells in fresh protein-free medium (e.g. PBS) to reduce background fluorescence.

3. Mix equal volumes (20–50 µl) of resuspended cells and dye solution, and leave at room temperature for 10 min.

4. Apply an aliquot to a microscope slide and cover with a coverslip.

5. Transfer the slide to the microscope, illuminate with appropriate filter, and count the cells (minimum of 500 for good sample size) that have either red or green fluorescent nuclei.

Notes

Acridine orange concentrations in the range 0.5–5 µmol l^{-1}, and propidium iodide concentrations in the range 50–100 µmol l^{-1} usually give good cell staining while avoiding intense background interference, but trial runs should be performed to optimize dye concentrations for particular cell type.

At concentrations above about 20 µmol l^{-1}, acridine orange also produces a red fluorescence following a metachromatic shift.

Protocol 1.15

Cell viability determined by protein synthesis

Equipment

Bench-top centrifuge

Pipets

Gas cylinder (95% O_2:5% CO_2)

Disposable plastic bottles (20 ml) and appropriate rubber bungs

Shaking water-bath at 37°C

Glass Pasteur pipets

Glass bottles (20 ml) with screw caps

Plastic trays with adsorbent paper lining

Scintillation vials

Scintillation counter

Pipets

Reagents

Krebs Ringer bicarbonate (KRB)

^{14}C-labeled L-leucine

Culture medium

Amino acid supplement for enhancing protein synthesis: e.g. Vamin, Vitrum (Sweden) at 5 ml per 100 ml KRB, or add 1 part full nutrient medium (e.g. Leibovitz L1 medium) to 4 parts KRB before use

Trichloroacetic acid (TCA) solution: 10% (w/v) in distilled water

NaOH solution: 20% (w/v) in distilled water

Solubilizing solution

Scintillation fluid

Protocol

1. Prepare the gassed KRB solution, and add trace quantities of [^{14}C]L-leucine (0.5 μCi/100 ml buffer gives adequate activity for hepatocyte studies).

2. Centrifuge the cell suspension. Discard supernatant. Resuspend the pellet in fresh protein-free culture medium, and count. Adjust the volume of medium as required (for hepatocytes 5–10 × 10^6 cells ml^{-1} are suitable).

3. Place sufficient plastic pots on ice and pipet into each 2 ml KRB containing [^{14}C]L-leucine and 0.5 ml cell suspension.

4. Blow O_2:CO_2 gas mixture on to the surface of the solutions for 1 min, and stopper tightly with rubber bungs.

5. Place the tubes in a shaking water-bath at 37°C, at a shaking speed of 50–80 cycles per min.

6. At time intervals, remove tubes, place on ice, and immediately add 5 ml cold 10% TCA. (For most studies 15-min intervals over 2 h are adequate.) Stand tubes on ice for 30 min.

7. At the end of the time course, pellet the precipitated proteins, and remove the supernatant. To each tube add 5 ml fresh 10% TCA. Agitate the tubes to resuspend the pellet, recentrifuge, and discard the supernatant.

8. Add 2 ml 1 M NaOH to each tube and stopper, stand in a water-bath at 70°C to dissolve the precipitate (2–3 h).

9. Transfer the dissolved proteins with glass Pasteur pipets into the glass bottles, add 5 ml 10% TCA, and stand on ice for 30 min.

10. Centrifuge the precipitated proteins and remove the supernatant. Allow the pellets to drain of moisture by inverting the bottles on blotting paper in plastic trays for a few hours.

11. Add 1 ml of solubilizing agent to each tube, tightly cap, and leave for several hours (or overnight).

12. Add between 50 and 100 µl of dissolved proteins to 10 ml scintillant solution in scintillation vials. Count in the scintillation counter using appropriate times and external/internal standards to correct for quench effects.

13. Relate incorporation of [^{14}C]leucine into protein over time per unit number of cells (derived from the original count).

Notes

Krebs Ringer bicarbonate (KRB). Make up stock solutions in (g/100 ml) distilled water as follows: (a) 0.9 g NaCl, (b) 1.15 g KCl, (c) 2.4 g $CaCl_2$ (hydrated), (d) 2.11 g KH_2PO_4, (e) 3.82 g $MgSO_4$ (hydrated), (f) 1.3 g $NaHCO_3$. Store the solutions in a fridge and combine when needed as follows: 100 parts (a), 4 parts (b), 5 parts (c), 1 part (d), 1 part (e), and 21 parts (f). Place the KRB on ice and gas for 20 min with 95% O_2:5% CO_2 before use.

Keep solutions on ice; protein synthesis will be inhibited until the samples are all warmed up together, and the solubility of the dissolved gas remains high.

The length of gassing in step 4 is sufficient for incubations of 2–3 h. Length of time is dependent on head space and so will vary with different volumes of suspension and volume of tubes.

The transfer to glass in step 9 is necessary because many of the solubilizing solutions will attack plastic tubes. The second dissolution/precipitation step also enhances purification of precipitated proteins from any residual free labeled amino acid.

See De Loecker et al. (1991).

Protocol 1.16

Cell viability determined by uptake of radiolabeled thymidine

Equipment

Laminar flow-hood

Hemocytometer

96-well tissue culture plates

Humidified tissue culture incubator with gaseous atmosphere set at 95% air:5% CO_2

Vacuum aspirator with sterile Pasteur pipets

Scintillation vials

Scintillation counter

Pipets

Reagents

DMEM with 0.4% (v/v) FBS

DMEM with 5% (v/v) FBS

Methyl[^{3}H]thymidine (aqueous solution, 1 mCi)

Dulbecco's PBS

TCA solution: 7.5% (w/v) in distilled water

NaOH solution and HCl solution; both 4% (w/v) in distilled water

Protocol

1. Isolate human vascular smooth cells (VSMC) and count using a hemocytometer. Plate at a concentration of 1–2000 cells/well in 200 µl DMEM plus 5% FBS. Culture for 24 h in the incubator to ensure cell attachment. Designate some wells as controls for assay of total DNA content.

2. Remove the supernatants by vacuum aspiration. Wash the wells with fresh pre-warmed DMEM, add 200 µl of DMEM containing 0.4% FBS and culture in the incubator for a further 24 h.

3. Aspirate supernatant, wash the wells with fresh pre-warmed DMEM. Add 200 µl DMEM plus 0.4% FBS to half the controls and half test wells. To the remainder add 200 µl DMEM plus 5% FBS. To all test wells, add 1 µCi of [^{3}H]thymidine.

4. Transfer the plates to the incubator for a further 24 h.

5. Aspirate supernatant. Wash the wells twice with pre-warmed PBS as before.

6. To the test wells add 200 µl 7.5% TCA. To the control wells add 200 µl PBS, dislodge the cells by scraping with a sterile pipet, harvest, and use for total DNA measurements. Place the plate on ice for 1 h to ensure precipitation of cell components.

7. Aspirate supernatant. Wash the wells with 200 µl fresh cold TCA, add 200 µl 4% NaOH, cover, and leave overnight at room temperature.

8. Remove the NaOH digests and add to 10 ml of scintillation fluid in scintillation vials. Wash each test well with 200 µl of 4% HCl and add this to the respective scintillation vial. Count the vials in a scintillation counter using appropriate times and external/internal standards to correct for quench effects.

9. Relate the incorporation of [³H]thymidine to DNA content of the control wells. Determine the replicative stimulus provided by exposure to high (5%) FBS.

Notes

Low cell numbers are plated initially to ensure sufficient surface area in the wells to allow continued growth over several days.

Total DNA may be assayed by a fluorimetric technique (Puzas and Goodman, 1978); pool the contents of two or more wells as there may be insufficient cell numbers in individual wells.

Culture in the presence of low FBS for VSMC induces quiescence and synchronizes the growth phase.

Measurement of thymidine incorporation in low (0.4%) and high (5%) FBS allows assessment of promotion of growth in a particular cell isolate and thus comparison between different VSMC preparations.

Protocol 1.17

Cell preparation by cytocentrifuge for immunostaining

Equipment

> Pipet
>
> Cytocentrifuge
>
> Filter cards
>
> Microscope slides

Reagents

> M199 culture medium containing 10% FBS

Protocol

> 1. Resuspend cells in M199 culture medium at a concentration of 1×10^6 cells ml^{-1}.
> 2. Mount the microscope slides in the cytocentrifuge with the filter papers.
> 3. To each of the wells add 100–300 µl of cell suspension.
> 4. Spin for 10 min at 45 *g*.
> 5. Remove the slides and leave the cytospins to air dry for up to 15 min at room temperature before proceeding further with immunostaining.

Notes

> Include positive and negative controls to ensure reagents react as expected when characterizing cells.
>
> Slides can be protected by wrapping in cling film and storing at −20°C for later use. If stored, it is necessary to leave the slides for up to 15 min at room temperature before unwrapping to avoid excessive ice recrystallization.

Protocol 1.18

Characterization of cells by indirect immunofluorescence staining

Equipment

Microscope slides

Wax pen

Coplin jar and slide rack

Pipet

Humidified chamber

Coverslips

Fluorescence microscope

Reagents

Fixative

PBS

Normal serum (e.g. swine serum)

Primary antibody

Secondary antibody (e.g. FITC-conjugated)

Bovine serum albumin (BSA, Fraction V)

Fluorescence mounting fluid

Protocol

1. Fix the cytospins in the chosen fixative for 10 min at room temperature.

2. Using a wax pen, circle around the edge of the cytospins. This prevents any running of the solution over the slides.

3. Wash gently in PBS for 5 min. Repeat wash with PBS. The slides can be left in PBS for the duration necessary.

4. Dilute the serum (1:20) in PBS containing 0.1% BSA.

5. To the cytospin, add 80 µl of the serum solution using a pipet.

6. Place in a humidified chamber and leave for 30 min.

7. Gently tap off the serum solution and add 80 µl of the primary antibody diluted (1:500) in PBS containing 0.1% BSA. Leave for 60 min in the humidified chamber.

8. Wash twice in PBS for 5 min, tapping off the excess fluid.

9. Add 80 µl of the secondary antibody diluted (1:40) in PBS containing 0.1% BSA. Leave in the humidified chamber for a further 60 min.

10. Wash twice in PBS for 5 min, tapping off the excess fluid.

11. Mount using fluorescent mounting fluid and cover with coverslip, avoid air bubbles.

12. Using phase-contrast microscopy locate cells and then view under epifluorescence. Positive cells will fluoresce green while negative cells show no fluorescence.

Notes

All steps are performed at room temperature.

Once cells have been fixed, do not let the slides dry out. The slides can be left in PBS.

After mounting, store slides in the dark at 4°C. The mounting medium prevents dehydration and photobleaching.

Photographs should be taken quickly and as soon as possible when checking for fluorescence.

For cell surface or particular fixation-sensitive antigens, treat with antibodies first, then fix. When cells are fixed after staining, incubations with antibody should be performed at 4°C to prevent internalization of antigen–antibody complexes.

Fixation renders cells resistant to mounting.

Immunofluorescent staining need not be performed *in situ* but can be performed in suspension. The method is essentially as described except smears or cytospins are prepared after staining.

Protocol 1.19

Indirect (DAB) immunoperoxidase staining

Equipment

Pipet

Microscope slides

Coplin jar and slide rack

Wax pen

Humidified chamber

Coverslips

Light microscope

Reagents

10% neutral-buffered formal saline

PBS

30% hydrogen peroxide

Primary antibody

Secondary antibody (e.g. HRP conjugated)

Human serum

DAB

Tris base

HCl

NaOH solution

Imidazole buffer

Counterstain (e.g. Mayer's Hemalum)

Mountant (e.g. Glycergel)

Protocol

1. Fix the prepared cytospins in formalin for 5 min at room temperature.

2. Gently wash in PBS for 5 min.

3. Using a wax pen, circle around the cytospins. This prevents any running of the solution over the slides.

4. Dilute hydrogen peroxide solution by adding 1.5 ml hydrogen peroxide to 50 ml PBS. Add a drop of this diluted hydrogen peroxide to the cytospin and leave for 15 min.

5. Wash twice in PBS for 5 min.

6. Add 80 µl of primary antibody diluted (1:40) in PBS containing 0.1% BSA. Leave for 60 min in a humidified chamber.

7. Gently tap off the antibody and wash twice in PBS for 5 min.

8. Add 80 µl diluted secondary antibody (1:60) in PBS containing 10% normal human serum. Leave for 60 min in the humidified chamber.

9. Prepare DAB solution: dissolve 0.608 g Tris base in 63 ml distilled water. Add 38 ml 0.1 M HCl and pH to 7.4–7.6 using either NaOH or HCl. To this add 60 mg DAB, 40 µl hydrogen peroxide and 1 ml 0.1 M imidazole.

10. Gently tap off the secondary antibody and wash with PBS for 5 min.

11. Immerse the slides in the DAB solution for 5 min.

12. Wash the slides with PBS for 5 min.

13. At this stage it is possible to counterstain with Mayer's Hemalum for 5 min.

14. Wash with PBS for 5 min.

15. Mount using Glycergel and cover with a coverslip, avoid air bubbles.

16. View using light microscopy. Positive cells will stain intense brown while negative cells and nuclei do not stain at all, unless counterstained.

Notes

DAB, 3′-diaminobenzidine tetrahydrochloride.

All steps are performed at room temperature.

Diluted hydrogen peroxide is used to quench the endogenous peroxidase activity.

It is important that DAB solution is made fresh for each procedure. Necessary precautions should be taken when using DAB as it is considered carcinogenic.

Prior to using DAB solution, take equal volumes (50 µl) of secondary antibody solution and DAB solution and mix. This should turn brown, if not then there has been an error in making up of one of the solutions.

Mayer's Hemalum is a nuclear stain, which will turn blue.

Protocol 1.20

Metabolic characterization of endothelial cells

Equipment

Pipet

Eight-chambered wells

5% CO_2 humidified incubator

Fluorescent microscope with a rhodamine excitation filter

Reagents

PBS without calcium and magnesium

0.1% gelatin (w/v) in PBS

Dil-acetylated low-density lipoprotein (LDL)

M199 culture medium containing FBS

3% formaldehyde

90% glycerol

Protocol

1. Prepare 0.1% gelatin in PBS and sterilize by autoclaving.

2. Coat the eight-chambered wells with 200 µl of 0.1% gelatin in PBS, and leave overnight at 37°C.

3. Plate separated endothelial cells onto the eight-chambered wells.

4. Place cells overnight in a 5% CO_2 incubator at 37°C and allow to grow until cells are semi-confluent.

5. Dilute dil-acetylated LDL to 10 µg ml^{-1} in M199 culture medium.

6. Add 300 µl of diluted dil-acetylated LDL to the cells and incubate for 4–6 h at 37°C in a CO_2 incubator.

7. Discard the media and wash cells with warm PBS. Repeat wash with PBS.

8. Using a fluorescent microscope with a rhodamine filter, check cells for positive red fluorescence.

9. Fix cell preparations using 3% formaldehyde in PBS for 20 min at room temperature.

10. Rinse cells with PBS.

11. Discard the fixative and mount slides with a drop of 90% glycerol and 10% PBS.

Notes

Protocol based on the method of Voyta *et al.* (1984).

Dil-acetylated LDL, acetylated LDL labeled with 1,1 dioctadecyl-1-3,3,3,3-teramethyl-indo-carbocyanine perchlorate.

Include positive and negative control cell suspensions in the procedure to ensure reagents react as expected.

Photographs should be taken quickly and as soon as possible when checking for fluorescence.

Do not use acetone or methanol fixation as dil-acetylated LDL is soluble in organic solvents.

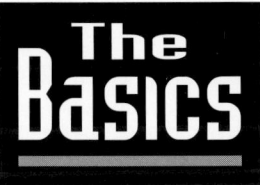

Chapter 2

Fractionation of cells by sedimentation methods

1. Introduction

One of the most common methods used for the separation of cells is sedimentation. A mixed population of cells may be separated into different cell types or subsets by virtue of their different sedimentation rates. The sedimentation rate of a cell in a medium is determined by cell size and/or cell density.

When cells are suspended in a medium they experience a force. The magnitude and direction of this force depends upon the effective size and density of the cells, the density and viscosity of the medium in which the cells are suspended, and the force field. In the case of unit gravity separations the force on the cells is that of the Earth's gravity (1 g) while, in centrifugation, the spinning rotor generates a centrifugal force that is dependent upon the speed of rotation and the distance from the axis of rotation. A greater force is experienced the further a particle is from the axis of rotation. The force exerted over a particle is called the relative centrifugal force (r.c.f.); it is expressed as multiples of the Earth's gravitational field "g" (e.g. 100 g). The r.c.f. generated by a spinning rotor is related to its speed of rotation in revolutions per minute (r.p.m.) and the distance of a particle from the axis in centimeters:

$$\text{r.c.f.} = 11.18 \times r \times (\text{r.p.m.}/1000)^2. \tag{2.1}$$

The speed required to achieve the required centrifugal force can be calculated:

$$\text{r.p.m.} = 299.07/\sqrt{\text{r.c.f.}/r} \tag{2.2}$$

where r is the distance of the particle from the center of rotation in centimeters.

The rate at which a particle migrates is described by the Stokes equation:

$$v = \frac{d^2(\rho_p - \rho_m)g}{18\mu} \tag{2.3}$$

where: v is the velocity of sedimentation (cm s^{-1}), d is the diameter of the particle (cm), ρ_p is the density of the particle (g cm^{-3}), ρ_m is the density of the medium (g cm^{-3}), g is the centrifugal force (dyne) and μ is the viscosity of the medium (poise).

From the Stokes equation it can be seen that:

1. the rate of particle sedimentation is proportional to the square of the size of the particle (d);

2. the sedimentation rate is proportional to the difference in density between the particle and the medium;

3. when the densities of the particle and medium are equal ($\rho_p - \rho_m = 0$), the particle stops migrating;

4. when the density of the medium exceeds that of the particle, the rate of sedimentation is negative, and the particle will migrate against the direction of the centrifugal force;

5. the sedimentation rate decreases as the liquid viscosity increases; and

6. the sedimentation rate increases as the gravitational force increases.

The equation also implies that cells can be separated either on the basis of their buoyant densities or on the basis of their sedimentation rates, the latter of which is determined primarily by differences in size. Centrifugal techniques that rely on differences in the sizes of cells are differential pelleting and rate-zonal centrifugation. Techniques relying upon density differences are isopycnic centrifugation and techniques using density barriers. A high degree of resolution of different types of cells can be obtained using rate-zonal, isopycnic and density-barrier methods whereas simple pelleting procedures, such as are involved in differential pelleting, can only give a limited resolution.

2.   Separation media

The separation of intact cell populations by sedimentation requires careful choice of the separation conditions. For example, animal cells are very sensitive to changes in their osmotic environments, taking up water and swelling in hypo-osmotic conditions, losing water and shrinking in hyperosmotic conditions. In extreme hypo-osmotic conditions, the swelling of the cells can be sufficient to lyse them, while, in general, cells are less liable to damage by hyper-osmotic environments. In either case, the changes in volume brought about by nonphysiological osmotic conditions result in changes in the buoyant densities of the cells. While such osmotic environments may not be optimal, small changes in buoyant density, induced by controlled changes in the osmolality of the separation medium, may sometimes be used to improve the resolution of some cells, which under normal physiological conditions would have close or similar buoyant densities. The ability to control the osmolality of gradients is an advantage for any gradient medium used for separating cells. As shown in Equation 2.3, the viscosity of a medium is also important in determining both the migration rates of cells in that medium and this in turn can affect the resolution of bands.

It is important that any medium used for cell separation meets the following requirements:

■ the medium should be nontoxic to the cells;
■ its presence should not affect the function or, morphology of the cells;
■ it should be easy to remove after fractionation;
■ the presence of the medium should not interfere with any subsequent assays;
■ a simple, efficient method of determining the density of the gradient solutions and gradient fractions is essential.

Table 2.1. Properties of gradient media used for separating cells

Medium	Molecular weight/size	Osmolality	Comments
Ficoll	400 000	Low at low concentrations	Can be toxic at high concentrations
Bovine serum albumin	68 000	Low–medium	High UV absorption
Percoll	Colloidal particles 15 nm diameter	Very low	Silica particles may stick to cells and be ingested
Metrizamide	789	Medium	High UV absorption
Nycodenz	821	Medium	High UV absorption
OptiPrep	1550	Low–medium	Dimeric structure reduces osmolality

There are few media that meet these requirements, as indicated in *Table 2.1*. Some solutes that are thought of as being relatively harmless can be toxic to cells. For example, while sucrose is widely used for organelle separations it tends to be toxic to intact cells and similarly salts that are used in balanced salt solutions can be toxic at higher concentrations.

While Percoll has become the most widely used medium for isopycnic cell separations, iodinated gradient media have also proved useful for both rate-zonal and isopycnic separations. The ionic, iodinated media, such as sodium metrizoate and sodium diatrizoate, were originally used for cell separations, but their osmolalities are relatively high and they can have toxic effects on cells. However, they are still widely used, very successfully, for some applications, notably for ready-prepared solutions for the routine separation of blood cells. The nonionic, iodinated media, metrizamide, Nycodenz and OptiPrep, have properties which come close to those of an ideal density gradient medium for cell separations; providing autoclavable, nontoxic and nonionic solutions of relatively high densities and low osmolality and ionic strength.

3.   Iso-osmotic gradients

As previously stated, when separating cells it is in most cases essential to use media that are iso-osmotic with the cells to be separated. In the case of animal cells that have no rigid cell walls it is essential that the osmolality is as close to physiological as possible as otherwise the cells can become damaged. However, in some cases, it is possible to deviate slightly from iso-osmotic conditions in order to optimize separations.

3.1   Percoll gradients

Percoll is the best known and most widely described of the colloidal silica media. It is supplied as a prepared suspension of 15-nm diameter silica particles coated with polyvinylpyrrolidone (PVP). The suspension supplied has density of 1.13 g ml^{-1} and osmolality of about 15–20 mOsm. The silica particles themselves do not contribute to the osmolality or the refractive index of the suspension, so the given osmolality and refractive index (1.3540) of the suspension is probably caused by free PVP. Iso-osmotic working solutions are prepared by adding solutions of culture medium, sodium chloride or glucose to the suspension. The working solutions will therefore have the osmolalities and refractive indices essentially determined by those of the diluent used. The colloidal nature of Percoll allows the formation of self-generated gradients in fixed-angle rotors using centrifugal forces of about 20 000–30 000 g for 30 min. Gradients form most quickly in vertical and shallow fixed-angle rotors; the use of swing-out rotors is not recommended. As the osmolality is almost entirely caused by the osmolality of the diluents, which do not sediment during centrifugation, the osmolality of the gradient can be maintained within narrow limits throughout.

The high ionic strengths of salt solutions increase the sedimentation rates of silica particles; thus shorter centrifugation times, or lower rotor speeds, are required to achieve the same density gradient, as compared with the nonionic (e.g. glucose) diluents. The reader should note that the density profiles of Percoll gradients will change continuously during centrifugation as the particles sediment; prolonged centrifugation at high speed will result in all the silica pelleting. This is not deemed a problem with gradients designed for cell separations, as the large size of the cells and their relatively rapid sedimentation rates require short centrifugation times and relatively low centrifugal forces.

The stock working suspensions of Percoll using NaCl as the osmotic balancer is prepared by mixing 1 volume of 1.5 M NaCl with 9 volumes of Percoll suspension (to obtain a refractive index of 1.3533 and density of 1.123 g ml^{-1}); 1.5 M NaCl has refractive index of 1.3475 and density of 1.06 g ml^{-1}. This stock working solution now contains 0.15 M NaCl and has an osmolality of about 290 mOsm. Dilution of this working solution to the densities required for iso-osmotic gradient formation is carried out using 0.15 M NaCl solutions (*Table 2.2*). The diluted fractions, using 0.15 M NaCl, are approximately 290 mOsm.

The density of the solutions can be calculated by:

$$(A \times \text{density of Percoll}) + (B \times \text{density of diluent}) / (A + B) \qquad (2.4)$$

where A is the number of parts of Percoll and B is the number of parts of diluent. Intermediate densities can be easily calculated.

The density of fractions from a Percoll gradient can best be determined by running an identical gradient, loaded with commercially available

Table 2.2. Colloidal silica media, Percoll, diluted with sodium chloride

Parts Percoll	Part diluent	Density (g ml^{-1})
1	9	1.018
2	8	1.029
3	7	1.041
4	6	1.053
5	5	1.065
6	4	1.076
7	3	1.088
8	2	1.100
9	1	1.111
10	0	1.123

density marker-beads in place of the sample. After fractionation of both gradients, the positions of the marker beads in each fraction indicate the density of the equivalent fraction of the sample gradient.

However there are a number of disadvantages to the use of Percoll gradients. First, while the suspension is sterile as supplied and stable to autoclaving, the suspension cannot be autoclaved once the tonicity of Percoll has been adjusted with osmotic balancers. Solutions used as diluents must be filtered or autoclaved separately before adding them to the Percoll stock solution. Another problem is caused by the adherence of silica particles to membranes, which prove difficult to remove even after several washes; multiple washes tend to damage the cells, causing reduced recovery of the cells of interest. Furthermore, the silica particles have been shown to be ingested by cells at temperatures above 5°C, producing artifactual bands. Finally, Percoll absorbs in the UV and is also incompatible with most protein assays.

3.2 Nonionic iodinated media

Metrizamide, Nycodenz and Optiprep (*Figure 2.1*) are routinely used for cell separation by sedimentation methods. Metrizamide and Nycodenz have very similar physical and chemical properties, the important difference being the absence of a sugar group on the Nycodenz molecule. In the absence of the sugar group, the presence of Nycodenz does not interfere with a number of the common chemical assays. Furthermore, Nycodenz solutions can be autoclaved while metrizamide cannot. Both metrizamide and Nycodenz solutions can provide iso-osmotic solutions (approximately 300 mOsm) for cell separations up to densities of 1.16 g ml^{-1}, sufficient to band most mammalian cells. Although Nycodenz does not interfere with most biochemical assays, it does interfere with Folin-phenol and microbiuret assays for protein, and the anthrone assay for polysaccharides. It also produces quenching of radiolabel scintillation. Nycodenz is available both in dry powder form or as a prepared solution of 27.6% (w/v) Nycodenz with osmolality of 295 mOsm, under the trade name Nycoprep 1.150.

Iodixanol is essentially a dimer of Nycodenz (Ford *et al.*, 1994) and is available only as a ready-to-use solution under the trade name OptiPrep. OptiPrep is a 60% (w/v) solution of Iodixanol, made up in water without any other additives. The OptiPrep solution as supplied has a density of 1.32 g ml^{-1} and osmolality of 260 mOsm. The low osmolality, combined with the high density, of OptiPrep, has widened the range of applications that can be carried out under iso-osmotic conditions, so that dense cells, such as mammalian sperm, can also be separated without exposing them to high osmotic environments.

The preparation of Nycodenz solution (and working solutions) from the dry powder is described in *Tables 2.3–2.5*. The inclusion of EDTA in the solution is necessary to stabilize the Nycodenz molecule during autoclaving. Tricine rather than Tris should be used for buffering solutions as the latter is toxic to some cells. Working solutions of OptiPrep are prepared from the stock solution using various diluents as shown in *Tables 2.6–2.10*. The diluent solutions are designed to maintain the osmolality of the diluted fractions.

For the purposes of cell separations, continuous gradients of the iodinated media cannot be self-generated.

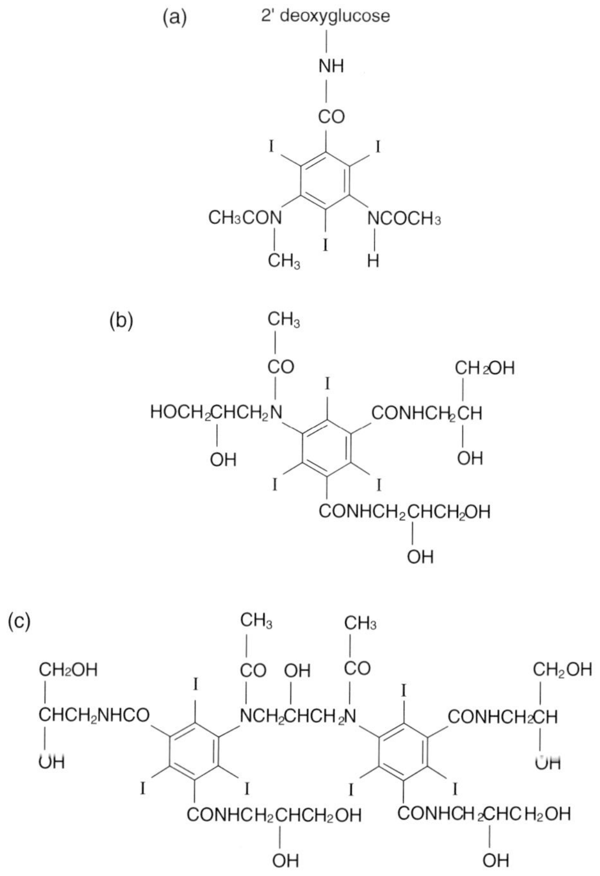

Figure 2.1

Iodinated gradient media, structures of (a) Metrizamide, (b) Nycodenz, and (c) Iodixanol (Optiprep).

Table 2.3. Composition of iso-osmotic Nycodenz solution

Solution	Constituent	Properties		
		Refractive index (20°C)	Density (g ml⁻¹)	Osmolality (mOsm)
Buffered medium	5 mM Tricine-NaOH (pH 7.5), 3 mM KCl, 0.3 mM CaEDTA	1.3332	—	20 ± 1
Nycodenz solution	27.6 g of solid Nycodenz dissolved and made up to 100 ml with buffered medium	1.3784	1.148 ± 0.002	290 ± 5
Sodium chloride diluent	0.75 g NaCl made up to 100 ml in the buffered medium	1.3345	1.003	250 ± 1
D-Glucose diluent	4.1 g D-glucose made up to 100 ml in the buffered medium	1.3449	1.014	250 ± 1

Table 2.4. Nycodenz diluted with sodium chloride

Parts Nycodenz	Parts diluent	Refractive index	Density (g ml⁻¹)
1	9	1.3389	1.017
2	8	1.3433	1.032
3	7	1.3477	1.046
4	6	1.3521	1.060
5	5	1.3564	1.074
6	4	1.3608	1.089
7	3	1.3652	1.103
8	2	1.3696	1.117
9	1	1.3740	1.132
10	0	1.3784	1.146

In Equation 2.5, $A=3.2574$ and $B=3.3440$.

Table 2.5. Nycodenz diluted with D-glucose

Parts Nycodenz	Parts diluent	Refractive index	Density (g ml⁻¹)
1	9	1.3483	1.027
2	8	1.3516	1.040
3	7	1.3549	1.054
4	6	1.3583	1.067
5	5	1.3616	1.080
6	4	1.3650	1.093
7	3	1.3684	1.106
8	2	1.3717	1.120
9	1	1.3750	1.133
10	0	1.3784	1.146

In Equation 2.5, $A=3.9403$ and $B=4.2853$.

Table 2.6. Diluent solutions for OptiPrep

Diluent	Preparation	Properties		
		Refractive index (20°C)	Density (g ml⁻¹)	Osmolality (mOsm)
Sodium chloride	0.8% (w/v) NaCl containing 20 mM Tricine/NaOH (pH 7.8)	1.3350	1.005	295
D-Glucose	4.4% (w/v) D-glucose containing 10 mM Tricine/NaOH (pH 7.8)	1.3398	1.015	270
Mannitol	4.4% (w/v) mannitol containing 10 mM Tricine/NaOH (pH 7.8)	1.3400	1.015	270
Sorbitol	4.4% (w/v) sorbitol containing 10 mM Tricine/NaOH (pH 7.8)	1.3398	1.014	265

Table 2.7. OptiPrep diluted with sodium chloride

Parts OptiPrep	Parts diluent	Refractive index	Density (g ml⁻¹)
1	9	1.3444	1.036
2	8	1.3537	1.068
3	7	1.3631	1.099
4	6	1.3725	1.131
5	5	1.3819	1.163
6	4	1.3912	1.194
7	3	1.4006	1.225
8	2	1.4100	1.257
9	1	1.4193	1.289
10	0	1.4287	1.320

In Equation 2.5, $A=3.3618$ and $B=3.4830$.

Table 2.8. OptiPrep diluted with D-glucose

Parts OptiPrep	Parts diluent	Refractive index	Density (g ml⁻¹)
1	9	1.3487	1.046
2	8	1.3576	1.076
3	7	1.3665	1.107
4	6	1.3754	1.137
5	5	1.3842	1.168
6	4	1.3931	1.198
7	3	1.4020	1.229
8	2	1.4109	1.259
9	1	1.4198	1.290
10	0	1.4287	1.320

In Equation 2.5, $A=3.4274$ and $B=3.5768$.

Table 2.9. OptiPrep diluted with mannitol

Parts OptiPrep	Parts diluent	Refractive index	Density (g ml⁻¹)
1	9	1.3487	1.045
2	8	1.3576	1.076
3	7	1.3665	1.106
4	6	1.3754	1.137
5	5	1.3842	1.167
6	4	1.3931	1.198
7	3	1.4020	1.228
8	2	1.4109	1.259
9	1	1.4198	1.289
10	0	1.4287	1.320

In Equation 2.5, $A=3.4353$ and $B=3.5880$.

Table 2.10. OptiPrep diluted with sorbitol

Parts OptiPrep	Parts diluent	Refractive index	Density (g ml⁻¹)
1	9	1.3487	1.044
2	8	1.3576	1.075
3	7	1.3665	1.106
4	6	1.3754	1.136
5	5	1.3842	1.167
6	4	1.3931	1.198
7	3	1.4020	1.228
8	2	1.4109	1.259
9	1	1.4198	1.289
10	0	1.4287	1.320

In Equation 2.5, $A=3.4443$ and $B=3.6009$.

A linear relationship between refractive index and the density of solutions of these media allows an equation to be derived from which the density of gradient fractions can be easily determined in the form;

$$\text{Density} = (\text{RI} \times A) - B \qquad (2.5)$$

where RI is the refractive index at 20°C and A and B are the derived constants.

Equation 2.5 is very accurate when the diluent is water, but less accurate when used with diluents containing salts and buffers, as the distribution of such salts changes with diffusion and their contribution to the refractive index can only be estimated. When buffers are used the following equation should be used:

$$\text{Refractive index (RI)} = \text{RI}_{\text{observed}} - (\text{RI}_{\text{buffer}} - \text{RI}_{\text{water}}). \qquad (2.6)$$

Yet, for practical, day to day purposes, it is possible to use the approximate constants for the diluents given, which should be sufficiently close and reproducible for most purposes.

3.3   Ficoll gradients

Ficoll (Ficoll 400), is a synthetic high-molecular-weight polymer (M_r=400 000) made by polymerization of sucrose with epichlorohydrin. Ficoll solutions can only be produced to give fairly narrow density ranges between 1.00 and 1.15 g ml⁻¹. Solutions below 20% (w/v) (1.07 g ml⁻¹) are osmotically inert but at concentrations above this there is a sharp increase in osmotic strength. Although the high viscous nature of Ficoll is not ideal for cell separation, the gradients are very stable. It is nontoxic to cells and does not interfere with most biological assays although some quenching of radiolabel scintillation counting can occur. Ficoll in aqueous solution is autoclavable but may caramelize if phosphate is present; in such cases Ficoll solutions may be sterilized by filtration or UV irradiation. Ficoll solutions need to be preformed into a gradient, they do not self-generate as Percoll does. The gradients produced are analyzed by measuring the refractive indices of the fractions, at 20°C. The density of the fractions can be determined using Equation 2.5, where the constants A and B are 2.381 and 2.175, respectively.

Removal of Ficoll from separated cells is best achieved by repeated washings. Although fibroblasts, hepatocytes, and tumor cells have been fractionated using Ficoll gradients (Castagna and Chauveau, 1969; Pretlow and Williams, 1973; Warters and Hofer, 1974), the high viscous and high osmotic nature of Ficoll solutions limits their use for cell separation. Combined with metrizoate or diatrizoate it has proven particularly useful for separating lymphocytes from whole blood where it is used primarily to aggregate the red blood cells (see Section 6).

3.4   Preparation of iso-osmotic gradients

Iso-osmotic density gradients can be prepared from any of media described using diluent solutions given for each medium. The colloidal silica media, such as Percoll, can provide useful preformed, self-generated, iso-osmotic gradients for cell separations, but can only be used for isopycnic separations. Preformed continuous or discontinuous iso-osmotic gradients of iodinated media can be prepared by a number of simple methods and they can be used for both rate-zonal and isopycnic separations.

Discontinuous iso-osmotic gradients

Discontinuous gradients are prepared simply by diluting a number of aliquots of a stock solution, with a suitable diluent, to the densities required and underlayering them into a centrifuge tube. The sample solution may be used as a diluent for one of the aliquots, thus the sample may be placed in the gradient in any position, top, middle or bottom. Once prepared, discontinuous gradients must be used immediately before significant diffusion, which smoothes out the interfaces, can take place.

Generally, a discontinuous gradient is only useful for isopycnic separations and in cases where the cell type of interest has a clear difference in buoyant density from the rest of the cells. The number of steps in the gradient, and the layer in which the sample is mixed, will depend upon the distributions of buoyant densities among the cell types present in the sample.

Continuous iso-osmotic gradients

For rate-zonal separations and where the cell type of interest has a buoyant density close to, or overlapping with, other cell types, a continuous gradient should be the gradient of choice. The density profile of a continuous gradient can be controlled to provide very shallow gradients within the density range required, in order to enhance the resolution of the bands of cells.

Continuous gradients can be prepared by one of two methods, by diffusion or mechanical gradient mixers (except for Percoll gradients, see earlier). Regardless of the method used to prepare a continuous gradient, the sample may be distributed throughout the gradient if one of the aliquots is diluted using the sample solution. Alternatively, after the gradient is formed, the sample can be mixed with the gradient medium to a final density a little denser than that of the bottom of the gradient. The sample may then be underlayered to the bottom of the gradient. The loading of samples within, or at the bottom of a gradient has the advantage of minimizing the formation of artifactual bands, that is, bands which contain trapped material which should have passed on to another banding area.

4. Choice of separation method

Cells may be separated by size using simple differential pelleting procedures or separated by virtue of their size and/or density using density gradient centrifugation. Nearly all cell separation procedures involve the pelleting of cells as part of the procedure for harvesting or concentrating cells prior to most fractionation procedures. However, differential pelleting is seldom used for separating different cell types, because the required difference in size, about 10-fold, is rarely seen and so this technique is not described in detail. Instead this chapter will concentrate on cell separations using density gradients with cells sedimenting in a centrifugal field. Aspects of cell separations that involve elutriation are described in Chapter 3.

The actual choice of technique will depend on the nature of the cell and the type of fractionation that is required. Cells are extremely diverse in terms of their morphologies but they can be broadly classified into two major groups: those with a rigid cell wall (e.g. bacterial, fungal and plant cells) and those without (e.g. animal cells and protoplasts). As previously mentioned, cells that do not possess a rigid cell wall are more difficult to fractionate because any significant variation in osmolality of the medium will cause the volume of the cell to change and so alter its sedimentation properties. Gradients that are used for osmotically sensitive cells should also be suitable for other types of cells although the presence of a rigid cell wall tends to make cells denser.

5. Separation of cells on the basis of size

Two methods of separation fall under this category, differential pelleting and rate-zonal separations. While both are limited in use, differential pelleting is described to some extent as it is often used as a first step in isolating enriched subpopulations. Rate-zonal centrifugation is briefly described but not discussed further.

Differential pelleting separates cells principally on the basis of size differences although differences in density can also be involved. The method involves allowing a homogeneous suspension of cells to sediment under the Earth's gravity or using low-speed centrifugation. The cells are suspended in a homogeneous, low density medium, usually an isotonic buffer or growth medium. Cells of different densities or size will sediment at different rates, the densest/largest sedimenting the fastest followed by less dense/smaller cells. As the medium used is homogeneous with respect to density, only two fractions are obtained, a pellet of cells at the bottom of the tube and cells in the supernatant (*Figure 2.2*). Note that the number of cells in the pellet for any given centrifugal force is dependent on their size and the time of centrifugation; if allowed to spin for long enough, all of the cells will collect in the pellet. Hence, the optimal time is that when the cells required are present largely in either the pellet or the supernatant. It should be possible to obtain a pure population of the smaller cells since these will remain largely uncontaminated in the supernatant after all of the larger cells have

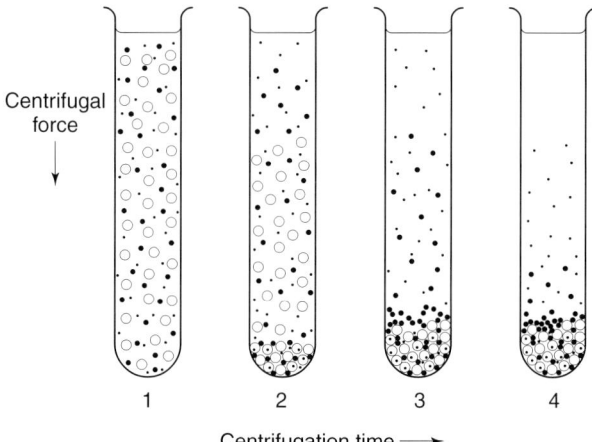

Centrifugal force ↓

1   2   3   4

Centrifugation time ⟶

Figure 2.2

Schematic diagram of differential pelleting of cells.

pelleted. However, it should be noted that the force required to pellet cells is also sufficient enough to pellet a proportion of the smaller cells.

Differential pelleting is seldom used for the isolation of cells of high purity due to the limitations described, however, one exception to this general rule is platelets: platelets are much smaller than other blood cells. Centrifugation of anticoagulated peripheral blood at 200 *g* for 10 min leaves the bulk of the platelets in the supernatant plasma, this separation can be improved by increasing the density of the medium (see Section 6).

Differential pelleting is often used as a first step in a separation procedure of several different cell types, for example, rat liver cells. The first step in the separation of these cells is to separate the parenchymal cells from the other (nonparenchymal) cells, see Section 6, by differential pelleting. Pelleting, resuspension and repelleting can give further enriched fractions but usually at the expense of yields and cell damage.

Again, this method is seldom used to obtain pure cell subpopulations but is used as a preparative step prior to further purification using isopycnic centrifugation (Section 6).

In rate-zonal centrifugation, the cells are centrifuged through a gradient the maximum density of which is less than that of the cells so that cells can continue to sediment until they reach the bottom of the tube, given sufficient time and speed of centrifugation. Rate-zonal separations are thus time dependent and use lower centrifugal forces than isopycnic separations. However, this method is limited by the tendency for cell clumping or aggregation experienced during separation, and so again, the preferred method of separation by sedimentation is that of separating cells on the basis of their density.

6.   Separation of cells on the basis of their density

Centrifugal separations of cells, principally on the basis of their density, has proven to be both an effective and economical way of obtaining pure populations. Cells with different buoyant densities can be separated on isopycnic density gradients. In isopycnic density centrifugation, the medium in which the cells are separated increases in density down the tube. Cells of a particular density sediment until they reach the point at which their density is the same as that of the gradient at which point they stop moving. The cells band according to their buoyant densities; the resolution of the bands will depend upon the degree of difference in the density profile of the gradient used.

Isopycnic centrifugation separates cells purely on the basis of differences in density. Differences in cell size merely affect the rates at which cells reach their equilibrium positions. An important point to note is that the equilibrium density of any particular cell type may vary when different density gradient media are used. This is because cells may become more or less hydrated depending on the medium used, which effectively alters their banding densities (Bøyum et al., 1983; Brouwer et al., 1992). Thus, for media such as Nycodenz, an osmotic balancer is required to maintain isotonic conditions necessary for osmotically sensitive mammalian cells.

The gradient used is either discontinuous (density-barrier) or continuous. Continuous gradients are ideal for the separation and characterization of cells. The continuous density gradient formed should cover the range of densities of the cells to be separated. The density at the bottom of the gradient is greater than the density of the densest cells to be separated such that the cells will never sediment to the bottom of the tube. The sample may be loaded at the bottom, top or mixed throughout the gradient. During centrifugation, cells migrate up or down the tube until they reach a point where the density of the medium is equal to the buoyant density of the cells (Figure 2.3). Isopycnic separations can be carried out either as unit gravity

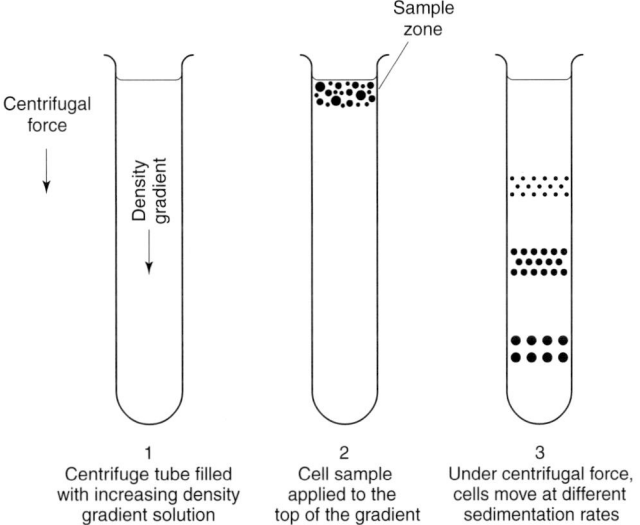

Figure 2.3

Schematic diagram of isopycnic separation of cells.

separations or by centrifugation. However, the sedimentation rate of cells in unit gravity is very slow particularly as cells approach their isopycnic positions (see Equation 2.3) and so isopycnic separations are almost always carried out using centrifugation to ensure that cells reach their isopycnic position in the gradient in a reasonably short time. An example of continuous isopycnic density centrifugation is that described by Ford and Rickwood (1983) for the separation of human leukocytes and red blood cells.

Once cells have been characterized, it is often more convenient to devise discontinuous gradients or density barrier methods for separating cells for routine or preparative purposes. In discontinuous gradients, single (one-step) or multiple (two-step, etc.) layers of medium of increasing density are used. The number of steps in the gradient, and the layer in which the sample is mixed, will depend upon the distributions of buoyant densities among the cell types present in the sample. The density at the bottom of the gradient may be less than the densest cells to be separated, allowing some cells to pellet.

6.1   Fractionation of blood cells using density-barrier methods

The diagnostic uses of human peripheral blood have meant that a number of methods have been developed to isolate the different cell types it contains. These usually involve the use of simple density barrier methods. Because of the routine nature of most of these cell separations, which are carried out in hospitals and clinics, ready-made solutions have been devised to enable many of these tasks to be carried out in a rapid and simple manner (*Table 2.11*).

One of the earliest, and still most widely used, method for isolating human mononuclear cells was that published by Bøyum (1968). The solution consists of a mixture of sodium metrizoate and Ficoll, which allowed the mononuclear cell fraction to be separated from the erythrocytes and polymorphonuclear cells. A number of other simple, routine methods of separating various types of blood cells have been devised since that first method was published.

Platelets

Platelets are small enucleated cells with functions related to blood-clotting. As a result of their small size, platelets will have slower sedimentation rates than the other peripheral blood cells. Simple differential centrifugation can be used to purify platelets but the yield is low. A higher yield is achieved by sedimenting the cells through a density barrier such that the erythrocytes and the nucleated cells are able to sediment rapidly through the medium, leaving the platelets to sediment slowly in a zone above them (*Protocol 2.1*). The platelets remain unactivated during fractionation and respond well to functional tests, such as aggregation studies.

Mononuclear cells

The mononuclear fraction of blood consists of lymphocytes, monocytes and basophils. The buoyant density of these cells in iso-osmotic conditions is significantly less than that of the other cell types, erythrocytes, neutrophils and eosinophils; this allows the use of a density-barrier type of separation using a layer of medium, dense enough to prevent the mononuclear

Table 2.11. Commercially available media for the isolation of different types of human peripheral blood cells

Medium	Composition (w/v)	Target cells	Supplier
Accu-prep	9.60% sodium metrizoate, 5.60% Ficoll	Mononuclear cells	Accurate Chemical
Histopaque 1077	9.60% sodium diatrizoate, 5.60% Ficoll	Mononuclear cells	Sigma
LSM	9.60% sodium diatrizoate, 5.60% Ficoll	Mononuclear cells	ICN
Lymphoprep	9.60% sodium metrizoate, 5.60% Ficoll	Mononuclear cells	Nycomed Amersham
1-step 1.077	14.10% Accudenz, 0.44% NaCl	Mononuclear cells	Accurate Chemical
1-step mixer	19.00% Accudenz, 0.20% NaCl	Mononuclear cells	Accurate Chemical
Nycoprep 1.077	14.10% Nycodenz, 0.44% NaCl	Mononuclear cells	Nycomed Amersham
Nycoprep mixer	19.00% Nycodenz, 0.20% NaCl	Mononuclear cells	Nycomed Amersham
1-step monocyte	13.00% Accudenz, 0.58% NaCl	Monocytes	Accurate Chemical
Nycoprep 1.068	13.00% Nycodenz, 0.58% NaCl	Monocytes	Nycomed Amersham
1-step polymorphs	13.80% sodium metrizoate, 8.00% dextran 500	Polymorphonuclear cells	Accurate Chemical
Histopaque 1119	16.70% sodium diatrizoate, 6.00% Ficoll	Polymorphonuclear cells	Sigma
Mono-poly resolving medium	15.50% sodium diatrizoate, 8.18% Ficoll	Polymorphonuclear cells	ICN
Polymorphprep	13.80% sodium metrizoate, 8.00% dextran 500	Polymorphonuclear cells	Nycomed Amersham
1-step platelets	12.00% Accudenz, 0.56% NaCl	Platelets	Accurate Chemical
Nycoprep 1.063	12.00% Nycodenz, 0.56% NaCl	Platelets	Nycomed Amersham

fraction passing through it, but allowing the other cells to pellet (*Protocols 2.2–2.4*).

Protocol 2.2 is the standard method of recovering the mononuclear fraction from human blood. It can also be used to recover mononuclear cells from disrupted spleen. However, as there are variations in the makeup and densities of blood cells from mammalian species other than human, the results obtained will vary between species. It may be necessary to vary the composition of the medium to obtain maximum recoveries.

Another solution and so protocol (*Protocol 2.3*) has been designed for the separation of the mononuclear fraction of blood; it avoids the necessity of layering the sample on top of the medium and is particularly suited to the isolation of mononuclear cells from large volumes of blood. In this method, the sample is mixed with an equal volume of the medium before centrifugation.

For a number of procedures it is desirable to separate the two major cell populations of the mononuclear fraction, the monocytes and lymphocytes. Monocytes can be separated from the bulk of the lymphocytes by taking advantage of the differential responses of the two types of cells to hypertonic conditions (*Protocol 2.4*). Ready-made media for the separation of monocytes from lymphocytes are available (*Table 2.11*). The monocyte separation described in *Protocol 2.4* does require some skill and experience in that the band of monocytes is not always very apparent because it is so diffuse.

Polymorphonuclear cells

The polymorphonuclear cells, neutrophils and eosinophils, are easily distinguished after staining by their lobed nuclei. Neutrophils make up the largest fraction of human leukocytes, about 45–70%. Unfortunately, the polymorphonuclear cells have banding densities, in iso-osmotic conditions, close to and overlapping with the erythrocytes. Still, they can be isolated, with varying degrees of purity and recovery, by a number of methods; one such method is described in *Protocol 2.5*. The method described works well because of the selected density, viscosity and osmolality of the solution. The density is much too high to allow passage of any of the cells in iso-osmotic conditions. The high osmolality causes the erythrocytes to lose water to the surrounding medium, thus they become denser and can sediment into the medium. The loss of water from the erythrocytes at the interface dilutes the medium generating a short density gradient, thus allowing the polymorphonuclear cells to migrate into this gradient. It is necessary to use undiluted blood in order that sufficient water is lost from the erythrocytes to form the gradient.

Erythrocytes

Although protocols described for isolating mononuclear cells can yield erythrocyte fractions (pellets), the cells are found to aggregate on resuspension because of the polysaccharides contained within the separation media. A method for the isolation of erythrocytes (red blood cells) is described in *Protocol 2.6*.

6.2   The purification of viable spermatozoa from bovine semen

Viable populations of spermatozoa, suitable for use in artificial insemination (AI), have been prepared from bovine ejaculates of poor quality, using either OptiPrep or Nycodenz solutions. Poor quality ejaculates, those containing a low percentage of normal, motile sperm and high percentages of dead or abnormal sperm, cannot be used for freezing and storing in aliquots for future AI. Using the techniques described in *Protocols 2.7* and *2.8*, the motile, normal populations from these ejaculates have been rescued and used successfully for AI. Both the described methods provide a band of motile, viable sperm in a condition suitable for freezing and using for artificial insemination, but there are some important differences.

In the Nycodenz method (*Protocol 2.7*), the cells are subjected to hyper-osmotic conditions, about 370–400 mOsm, which although it does not seem to affect the viability of the cells, does affect their banding densities (Bendixen and Rickwood, 1994). Keeping the osmolality as low as possible means that the sample material has to be loaded in the middle of the gradient, with the motile and the dead cells sedimenting. As a result of the high concentration of cells necessary in the loading area, during sedimentation, the mass of dead cells tends to sweep up a number of motile cells as they pellet, and the mass of motile cells at the interface tends to trap a number of dead cells within the band. The ability to load the ejaculate under iso-osmotic conditions at the bottom of the gradient when using the OptiPrep method (*Protocol 2.8*) minimizes this artifactual banding, resulting in a higher recovery of the viable fraction in a highly purified state, generally better than 96% viable, while the Nycodenz method gives a slightly lower recovery (80–85% viable cells) at a lower concentration.

It has been found that ejaculates from other mammalian species such as human, horse, pig and goat can be separated by the method described, but that some adjustment to the gradient densities and diluent solutions may be required depending on the species.

6.3   The separation of viable and nonviable cells from disaggregated tissue and lavages

Cell suspensions obtained by enzymic digestion of tissue and lavages of body cavities, can present difficulties caused by the debris from cells broken open during the digestion or lavaging procedure. The macromolecular contents spilled from these damaged cells, into the suspending medium, especially DNA, cause sticky aggregates to form during centrifugation. Thus, attempts to separate bands of cells on a density gradient can be frustrated by the presence of long, stringy aggregates throughout the gradient. This not only significantly reduces the recovery of cells from the bands, it can also prevent satisfactory fractionation of the gradients.

The nonionic, iodinated media offer a method to avoid such difficulties, and also to minimize the damage that can be caused when concentrating the cells by pelleting them. In metrizamide, Nycodenz and OptiPrep solutions damaged cells assume a higher density than the intact cells. Under iso-osmotic conditions, all intact mammalian cells have been found to have buoyant densities of less than 1.12 g ml^{-1} (with the exception of spermatozoa). If a cell suspension is spun down on to a cushion of one of these media, with a density of 1.15 g ml^{-1}, the intact cells will stop at the interface, while the damaged cells will sediment through the medium and pellet (*Protocol 2.9*). Most of the cytoplasmic contents of broken cells, which have spilled into the suspension, will remain in the supernatant. This will allow the band of intact cells at the interface of the suspension and medium, to be harvested in a concentrated form, while leaving most of the potentially interfering DNA in the supernatant. The recovered cells can then be separated on a density gradient much more readily.

6.4   The fractionation of cells from disaggregated rat liver

The single-cell suspension, obtained by perfusion of the whole liver *in situ*, will contain a variety of cell types; the greatest proportion (60%) will consist of parenchymal cells, also called hepatocytes. The other cells (nonparenchymal cells) consist primarily of sinusoidal cells, which in turn are composed of endothelial cells (15%), stellate or fat-storing cells (10%) and macrophages (10%), known as Kupffer cells. The percentages account for the proportion of cells of total liver cells. The hepatocytes are significantly larger than the nonparenchymal cells.

From a single rat liver, the suspension of single cells is usually contained in a volume of about 50 ml of incubation medium. The viable cells are concentrated while removing the dead cells and macromolecular species by following *Protocol 2.9*. The subsequent steps will depend upon the cell population of interest, whether it is the hepatocytes or the nonparenchymal cells that are required. *Protocol 2.10* describes the separation of rat liver cells using continuous Percoll gradients.

Alternatively, differential pelleting of cells harvested in *Protocol 2.9*, gives an almost pure suspension of parenchymal cells (hepatocytes); this is possible because of their very large size as compared with the nonparenchymal cells (*Protocol 2.11*).

The supernatants saved after spinning down the hepatocytes (from *Protocol 2.11*) will of course be enriched with nonparenchymal cells at low cell concentration in a relatively large volume. The cells may be concentrated as described in *Protocol 2.9*; however, the supernatant will be contaminated with some parenchymal cells which can be removed by repeated centrifugation at 600 *g* for 4 min at 4°C. The separation of the three populations of nonparenchymal cells can cause some difficulty as their buoyant densities tend to overlap. The yield of nonparenchymal cells obtained is, however, low due mainly to the repeated centrifugation steps. *Protocol 2.12* describes the separation of liver sinusoidal cells on Nycodenz gradients.

The Kupffer and endothelial cells of the normal rat liver cannot be completely purified by isopycnic density centrifugation alone. Knook *et al.* (1977) have shown that the density separation of these cell types can be improved by preloading of the Kupffer cell population with Jectofer® (an iron complex) *in vivo*. After this treatment the density distribution of Kupffer cells is shifted towards higher densities and relatively pure fractions of each cell type can be obtained.

6.5   Isolation of protoplasts from digested plant tissue

Once cellulose walls have been removed from plant cells, the plant cells become sensitive to osmotic changes in the environment, shrinking or swelling and thus varying in their buoyant densities. Hence, using density gradients to purify the intact protoplasts from the digest of debris from the digested walls and broken protoplasts, requires attention to the osmotic strength of the gradient medium.

The osmolality of the digest medium is obviously of importance; Sarhan and Cesar (1988) suggested that determining the osmolality of the living plant tissue and using a digest mixture of 1.8 times that measurement gave good results. This procedure is followed in *Protocol 2.13*, with the osmolality of the gradient solutions also set to that osmolality. Other methods for isolation of protoplasts using sedimentation are described in Dixon and Gonzales (1994).

6.6   Enhanced isopycnic separation of cells by density perturbation

Isopycnic density centrifugation is limited by the differences in density of different cell types. Within a homogeneous population of a particular type of cell, there exists a heterogeneity in cell density (Pretlow and Pretlow, 1982). Furthermore, heterogeneity exists within a single cell population, such as in the position of cells in the cell cycle (Pardee, 1989), or the presence of multiple cell types in the population as a result of cell differentiation (Childs *et al.*, 1983). The latter have been found to express different cell surface antigens (Swann *et al.*, 1992). However, a variety of approaches have been developed for modifying selectively the density of cells and subcellular components.

As previously mentioned, the buoyant densities of lymphocytes and monocytes overlap and so create problems when requiring highly purified lymphocytes. A procedure to overcome this uses the ability of monocytes to engulf colloidal iron particles when incubated *in vitro*. Their density can be increased sufficiently to allow them to sediment through the medium with the erythrocytes and granulocytes, leaving the lymphocytes at the interface (Bøyum, 1976).

Further density perturbation methods include those of Ghetie *et al.* (1974; 1975). They designed a cell separation technique based on the interaction between cell surface bound IgG and protein A of *Staphylococcus aureus*. The density of lymphoid cells coated with IgG antibodies against one of the surface markers was increased by adherence of staphylococci. Cells with adhering bacteria were separated from cells without bacteria by density gradient centrifugation (Ghetie *et al.*, 1974). Alternatively, lymphocytes were incubated with sheep erythrocytes coated with protein A of *S. aureus*. Rosettes (complex of cells bound to target cell) were formed which were then separated from nonrosetted lymphocytes by density gradient centrifugation (Ghetie *et al.*, 1975). Many other lymphocyte rosetting techniques and gradient separations exist (Albrechtsen *et al.*, 1977; Galili and Schlesinger, 1974; Parish *et al.*, 1974; Pellegrino *et al.*, 1976).

Another density perturbation procedure for the fractionation of cells (Patel and Rickwood, 1995; Patel *et al.*, 1993; 1995) is also described. Cells were labeled with antibody-coated dense beads and then fractionated on isotonic isopycnic OptiPrep gradients (*Protocol 2.14*). Cells that had not bound the dense beads were recovered from the top of the gradient while cells associated with the dense beads were found in progressively denser regions of the gradient. Unlabeled cells could be separated from labeled cells. Cells were labeled via antigen-antibody specificity, allowing the isolation of immunologically distinct subpopulations. A typical separation that can be achieved using the density perturbation method described is shown in *Figure 2.4*. It shows the fractionation of a culture of MOLT-4 cells into immunologically different subpopulations.

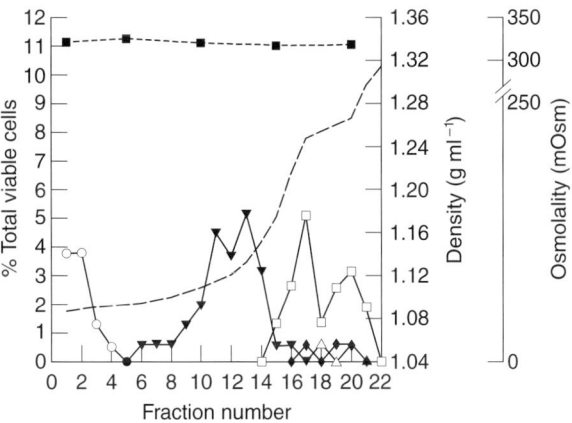

Figure 2.4

Fractionation of cells using density perturbation methods. Tissue culture (MOLT-4) cells were mixed with antibody-coated Dynabeads and separated on an isopycnic continuous OptiPrep gradient. (O) cells without beads bound; (▼) cells with 1–3 beads bound; (❑) cells with 7–9 beads bound; (◆) cells with 13–15 beads bound; (△) cells with 19+ beads bound; (—) density, g ml⁻¹; and (■) osmolality, mOsm.

7.   Concluding remarks

The described sedimentation methods make it is possible to separate cells which are similar in buoyant density and to separate cells with high purity. They offer a wide range of techniques for separating viable cells from all types of organisms, and are particularly useful when the required through-put is large. The methods can in some cases be modified; for example iso-pycnic separations can be enhanced by density perturbation methods as described.

References

Albrechtsen, D., Solheim, B.G. and Thorsby, E. (1977) Serological identification of five HLA-D associated (Ia-like) determinants. *Tissue Antigens* 9: 153–162.

Bendixen, B. and Rickwood, D. (1994) Properties and applications of a new type of iodinated gradient medium. *J. Biochem. Biophys. Methods* 28: 43–52.

Bøyum, A. (1968) Isolation of mononuclear cells and granulocytes from human blood. Isolation of mononuclear cells by one centrifugation, and of granulo-cytes by combining centrifugation and sedimentation at 1g. *Scand. J. Clin. Lab. Invest.* 21: 77–89.

Bøyum, A. (1976) Isolation of lymphocytes, granulocytes and macrophages. *Scand. J. Immunol.* 5: 9–15.

Bøyum, A., Berg, T. and Blomhoff, R. (1983) Fractionation of mammalian cells. In *Iodinated Density Gradient Media: A Pratical Approach* (ed. D. Rickwood). IRL Press, Oxford, pp. 147–171.

Brouwer, A., Hendriks, H.F.J., Ford, T. and Knook, D.L. (1992) Centrifugation sep-arations of mammalian cells. In *Preparative Centrifugation: A Practical Approach* (ed. D. Rickwood). IRL Press, Oxford, pp. 271–314.

Castagna, M. and Chauveau, J. (1969) Separation of metabolically distinct cell frac-tions from isolated rat hepatocyte. *Exp. Cell Res.* 57: 211–212.

Childs, R.A., Pennington, J., Uemure, K., Scudder, P., Goodfellow, P.N., Evans, M.J., and Feizi, T. (1983) High-molecular-weight glycoproteins are the major carriers of the carbohydrate differentiation antigens I, i and SSEA of mouse ter-atocarinoma cells. *Biochem. J.* 215: 491–503.

Dixon, R.A. and Gonzales, R.A. (eds) (1994) *Plant Cell Culture, A Practical Approach*, 2nd edn. IRL Press at Oxford University Press, Oxford.

Ford, T.C. and Rickwood, D. (1983) The separation of cells on iso-osmotic Nycodenz gradients. *Biochem. Soc. Trans.* 11: 273.

Ford, T.C. and Rickwood, D. (1990) A new one-step method for the isolation of human mononuclear cells. *J. Immunol. Methods* 134: 237–241.

Ford, T.C. and Rickwood, D. (1992) Improved isolation of mononuclear cells from stored blood. *Clin. Chim. Acta* 206: 249–252.

Ford, T.C., Graham, J. and Rickwood, D. (1990) A new, rapid, one-step method for the isolation of platelets from human blood. *Clin. Chim. Acta* 192: 115–120.

Ford, T., Graham, J. and Rickwood, D. (1994) Iodixanol: a nonionic iso-osmotic centrifugation medium for the formation of self-generated gradients. *Anal. Biochem.* 220: 360–366.

Galili, U., and Schlesinger, M. (1974) The formation of stable E rosettes after neur-aminidase treatment of either human peripheral blood lymphocytes or of sheep red blood cells. *J. Immunol.* 112: 1628–1634.

Ghetie, V., Nilsson, K. and Sjöquist, J. (1974) Density gradient separation of lym-phoid cells adhering to protein-A-containing Staphylococci. *Proc. Natl Acad. Sci. USA* 71: 4831–4835.

Ghetie, V., Stålenheim, G. and Sjöquist, J. (1975) Cell separation by staphylococcal protein A-coated erythrocytes. *Scand. J. Immunol.* 4: 471–477.

Knook, D.L., Blansjaar, N. and Sleyster, E.Ch. (1977) Isolation and characterization of Kupffer and endothelial cells from the rat liver. *Exp. Cell Res.* 109: 317–329.

Pardee, A.B. (1989) G_1 events and regulation of cell proliferation. *Science* **246**: 603–608.

Parish, C.R., Kirov, S.M., Bowern, N. and Blanden, R.V. (1974) A one-step procedure for separating mouse T and B lymphocytes. *Eur. J. Immunol.* **4**: 808–815.

Patel, D. and Rickwood D. (1995) Optimization of conditions for specific binding of antibody-coated beads to cells. *J. Immunol. Methods* **184**: 71–80.

Patel, D., Rubbi, C.P. and Rickwood, D. (1993) Use of density perturbation to isolate immunologically distinct populations of cells. *J. Immunol. Methods* **163**: 241–251.

Patel, D., Rubbi, C.P. and Rickwood, D. (1995) Separation of T and B lymphocytes from human peripheral blood mononuclear cells using density perturbation methods. *Clin. Chim. Acta* **240**: 187–193.

Pellegrino, M.A., Ferrone, S. and Theofilopoulos, A.N. (1976) Isolation of human T and B lymphocytes by rosette formation with 2-aminoethylisothiouronium bromide (AET)-treated sheep red blood cells and with monkey red blood cells. *J. Immunol. Methods* **11**: 273–279.

Pertoft, H., Rubin, K., Kjellen, L., Laurent, T.C. and Klingeborn, B. (1977) The viability of cells grown or centrifuged in a new density gradient medium, Percoll. *Exp. Cell Res.* **110**: 449–457.

Pretlow, T.G. and Williams, E.E. (1973) Separation of hepatocytes from suspensions of mouse liver cells using programmed gradient sedimentation in gradients of Ficoll in tissue culture medium. *Anal. Biochem.* **55**: 114–122.

Pretlow, T.G., II, and Pretlow, T.P. (1982) Sedimentation of cells: an overview and discussion of artifacts. In *Cell Separation: Methods and Selected Applications*, Vol. 1 (eds T.G. Pretlow II and T.P. Pretlow). Academic Press, New York, pp. 41–60.

Sarhan, F. and Cesar, D. (1988) High-yield isolation of mesophyll protoplasts from wheat, barley and rye. *Physiologia Plantarum* **72**: 337–342.

Swann, I.D., Dealtry, G.B. and Rickwood, D. (1992) Differentiation-related changes in quantitative binding of immunomagnetic beads. *J. Immunol. Methods* **152**: 245–251.

Warters, R.L. and Hofer, K.G. (1974) The *in vivo* reproductive potential of density separated cells. *Exp. Cell Res.* **87**: 143–151.

Protocol 2.1

Isolation of platelets from human peripheral blood (Ford *et al.*, 1990)

Equipment

Bench-top refrigerated centrifuge with swinging-bucket rotor

Centrifuge tubes

Pasteur pipets

Reagents

Separating medium: 12% (w/v) Nycodenz made up in 0.56% (w/v) NaCl solution, containing 5 mM Tricine/NaOH pH 7.0 (solution has density 1.063 g ml^{-1} and osmolality 320 mOsm)

Freshly drawn blood with sodium citrate as the anticoagulant

Protocol

1. Overlayer 5 ml freshly drawn blood carefully on top of 5 ml medium in a 10–15-ml centrifuge tube.

2. Centrifuge in a swinging-bucket rotor, at 350 **g** for 12–15 min at 20°C.

3. The platelets will be distributed from the sample/medium interface, into the medium. A fairly prominent band should occupy the first 1.0–1.5 cm, gradually diffusing towards the pellet. Harvest platelets from this band.

Notes

Alternatively, ready made separating media can be purchased, e.g. Nycoprep 1.063, see *Table 2.11* for details.

Keep blood samples and medium at 20°C and also centrifuge at this temperature.

After centrifugation, a pellet of erythrocytes will be found, with the nucleated cells laying on top of the pellet in the form of a 'buffy coat'.

About 70% of the platelet population can be recovered in the prominent band, with less than 1% contamination by other cells. By continuing to harvest platelets further towards the pellet of erythrocytes, about 95% of the platelets can be recovered, but, the closer to the pellet, the greater the contamination by other cells.

Protocol 2.2

The isolation of mononuclear cells from diluted blood (Bøyum, 1968)

Equipment

Bench-top refrigerated centrifuge with swinging-bucket rotor

Centrifuge tubes

Pasteur pipets

Reagents

Separating medium: 9.6% (w/v) sodium metrizoate or sodium diatrizoate, and 11% (w/v) polysaccharide (Ficoll 400 or Dextran 500) (solution has density 1.077 g ml^{-1} and osmolality 290 mOsm)

Blood samples, with any of the standard anticoagulants

0.9% (w/v) NaCl

Protocol

1. Mix the whole blood with an equal volume of 0.9% (w/v) NaCl.

2. Layer the diluted blood on top of the separating medium in a suitable centrifuge tube, in the ratio of 3.0 ml medium to 6–7 ml of the diluted blood.

3. Centrifuge at 800 *g* for 20 min at 20°C.

4. Harvest the band of mononuclear cells found at the sample/medium interface.

Notes

Alternatively, ready made separating media can be purchased, e.g. Lymphoprep, see *Table 2.11* for details.

There may be variation of the recovery rates depending upon the type of anticoagulant used.

Protocol 2.3

The isolation of mononuclear cells from whole blood (Ford and Rickwood, 1990; 1992)

Equipment

Bench-top refrigerated centrifuge with swinging-bucket rotor

Centrifuge tubes

Pasteur pipets

Reagents

Separation medium: 19% (w/v) Nycodenz in 0.2% (w/v) NaCl, 5 mM

Tricine/NaOH pH 7.4 (solution has density 1.10 ± 0.001 g ml^{-1} and osmolality 275 ± 15 mOsm)

Blood samples, with any of the standard anticoagulants

Protocol

1. Mix the whole blood with an equal volume of the medium by inverting the tube several times.

2. Place the mixture in a suitable size centrifuge tube and centrifuge at 800–1000 *g* for 30 min at 20°C.

3. Harvest the mononuclear cells from the top 1.5–2.0 cm of the gradient, making sure to collect all cells around the meniscus.

Note

Alternatively, ready made separating media can be purchased, e.g. Nycoprep Mixer, see *Table 2.11* for details.

Protocol 2.4

The fractionation of human mononuclear cells (Bøyum, 1983)

Equipment

Bench-top refrigerated centrifuge with swinging-bucket rotor

Centrifuge tubes

Pasteur pipets

Reagents

Separation medium: 13% (w/v) Nycodenz in 0.58% (w/v) NaCl, 5 mM Tricine/NaOH pH 7.4 (solution has density 1.068 ± 0.001 g ml^{-1} and osmolality 335 ± 5 mOsm)

Blood samples, with any of the standard anticoagulants

Protocol

1. Allow the blood (3–5 ml) containing anticoagulant to sediment at room temperature, the actual time required is quite variable depending on the source. Alternatively, the blood can be centrifuged at 200 **g** for 10 min.

2. On top of the pelleted erythrocytes a white top layer will be observed which is called the 'buffy coat'. Using a Pasteur pipet carefully remove as much of the buffy coat layer as possible to give a volume of about 3 ml of leukocyte-rich plasma and place in a 12-ml centrifuge tube.

3. Carefully underlayer the cell suspension with 3 ml of the separating medium and centrifuge at 600 **g** for 15 min at 20°C.

4. The monocyte layer will be seen as a very diffuse, gray band of turbidity centered around the position of the interface. Remove this band using a Pasteur pipet, immunological staining should show that the population is more than 90% monocytes.

Note

Alternatively, ready made separating media can be purchased, e.g. Nycoprep 1.068, see *Table 2.11* for details.

Protocol 2.5

The isolation of polymorphonuclear cells from blood

Equipment

Bench-top refrigerated centrifuge with swinging-bucket rotor

Centrifuge tubes

Pasteur pipets

Reagents

Separation medium: 13.8% sodium metrizoate and 8% Ficoll 400 or Dextran 500 (solution has density 1.113 ± 0.001 g ml^{-1} and osmolality 460 ± 15 mOsm)

Freshly drawn (less than 4 h) human blood

Protocol

1. Place 5.0 ml of the medium into a 12–15-ml centrifuge tube and layer 5.0 ml of the undiluted blood on top.

2. Centrifuge at 500 **g** for 30–35 min at 20°C.

3. After centrifugation, two bands of leukocytes will be found, one at the sample/medium interface, and one about 1 cm below it. The top band is of mononuclear cells, and the lower band consists of neutrophils, together with a few eosinophils that are separated on a rate-zonal basis. The erythrocytes are pelleted. Harvest polymorphonuclear cells.

Notes

Use whole, undiluted blood, anticoagulated with EDTA, heparin or citrate.

Use freshly drawn (less than 4 h) blood.

If the separation between the two leukocyte bands is greater or less than required then the length of time of centrifugation must be adjusted.

Temperature affects the separation; if the temperatures of the solutions or centrifuge are higher than 20°C then the time of centrifugation must be shortened.

If only 3.0 ml of whole blood is used, a similar separation takes place, but the separation of the two leukocyte bands is less than 0.5 cm, making them difficult to harvest without cross contamination. The gradients can be scaled up, using for example, 20 ml of blood and 10 ml of medium in a centrifuge tube that allows the column heights to be approximately the same as in the smaller version.

Protocol 2.6

Isolation of erythrocytes

Equipment

        Bench-top centrifuge

        Centrifuge tubes

        Pasteur pipets

Reagents

        Separating medium, Nycoprep 1.150 (Nycomed Amersham)

        Isotonic phosphate-buffered saline (PBS)

        3.8% trisodium citrate solution in water

Protocol

1. Mix 9 ml blood with 1 ml 3.8% trisodium citrate solution.

2. Centrifuge at 100 **g** for 30 min to sediment the erythrocytes.

3. Discard the supernatant and the top 2 mm of the pellet, which will contain platelets and white blood cells.

4. Prepare solution A by mixing one part Nycoprep 1.150 and one part PBS.

5. Prepare solution B by mixing one part Nycoprep 1.150 and one part solution A.

6. Prepare solution C by mixing two parts solution A and one part solution B.

7. Prepare solution D by mixing one part solution A and two parts solution B.

8. Add 1.5 ml solution A to a centrifuge tube. Underlayer with 1.5 ml solution C. Next underlayer with 1.5 ml solution D. Lastly, underlayer with 1.5 ml solution B. This yields a discontinuous gradient with the least dense at the top of the centrifuge tube and the most dense at the bottom.

9. Carefully apply 0.25 ml of the packed erythrocytes on to the top of the gradient.

10. Centrifuge at 500 **g** for 30 min at room temperature.

11. Harvest the erythrocytes banded at each interface layer. Each band represents erythrocytes of differing ages, the older cells being more dense and so banding at higher buoyant densities than younger cells.

12. Wash harvested cells in PBS.

Protocol 2.7

The isolation of viable spermatozoa from bovine semen using Nycodenz gradients

---

Equipment

Bench-top refrigerated centrifuge with swinging-bucket rotor

Centrifuge tubes

Pasteur pipets

Reagents

40% (w/v) Nycodenz solution made up in distilled water

Diluent solution; 11.65 g tri-sodium citrate, 1.75 g sodium hydrogen carbonate, 5.5 g Tris base, 2.35 g Na$_2$EDTA, 4.1 g citric acid, 1.0 g lincospectin, 0.75 g potassium chloride, 1.0 g polyvinyl alcohol, 70 mg cysteine, 16 g sorbitol, pH 7.0; made up to 1 l in glass-distilled water

Freshly taken bovine ejaculate

Protocol

1. Dilute an aliquot of the stock Nycodenz solution to 35% (w/v), using the diluent solution.

2. Mix a freshly taken, undiluted bovine ejaculate with an equal volume of the stock 40% Nycodenz.

3. Place the sample/Nycodenz mixture into a centrifuge tube and underlayer with the 35% Nycodenz aliquot.

4. Centrifuge at 1500 **g** for 25 min at 20°C in a swinging-bucket rotor.

5. After centrifugation, harvest the band of viable, motile cells of normal morphology found at the 35%/40% interface.

Note

The pelleted material consists of dead cells and a band of material at the top of the gradient consists of deformed cells and detached cytoplasmic droplets.

Protocol 2.8

The isolation of viable spermatozoa from bovine semen using OptiPrep gradients

Equipment

Bench-top refrigerated centrifuge with swinging-bucket rotor

Centrifuge tubes

Pasteur pipets

Reagents

OptiPrep solution

Diluent solution; 11.65 g tri-sodium citrate, 1.75 g sodium hydrogen carbonate, 5.5 g Tris base, 2.35 g Na_2EDTA, 4.1 g citric acid, 1.0 g lincospectin, 0.75 g potassium chloride, 1.0 g polyvinyl alcohol, 70 mg cysteine, 16 g sorbitol, pH 7.0; made up to 1 l in glass-distilled water

Freshly taken bovine ejaculate

Protocol

1. Dilute aliquots of OptiPrep with the diluent solution to final densities of 1.11 g ml^{-1} (1 part OptiPrep to 2 parts diluent) and 1.13 g ml^{-1} (5 parts OptiPrep to 7 parts diluent).

2. Mix a freshly taken, undiluted ejaculate with an equal volume of stock OptiPrep, to give a final density of approximately 1.17 g ml^{-1}.

3. Prepare a discontinuous gradient by underlayering the aliquots of OptiPrep into a centrifuge tube, 1.11 g ml^{-1} first, followed by the 1.13 g ml^{-1} aliquot and finally the sample/OptiPrep mixture.

4. Centrifuge the gradient at 1500 *g* for 25 min at 20°C in a swinging-bucket rotor.

5. After centrifugation, harvest the band of viable, motile cells of normal morphology found at the 1.11/1.13 g ml^{-1} interface.

Note

A pellet and particulate material consisting of dead cells remains in the loading area and a rather diffuse band of deformed cells and detached cytoplasmic droplets is found at the top of the gradient.

Protocol 2.9

Purification and enrichment of viable cells prior to further fractionation

Equipment

Bench-top refrigerated centrifuge with swinging-bucket rotor

Centrifuge tubes

Pasteur pipets

Reagents

Stock solution of one of the nonionic, iodinated density gradient media

Suitable diluent solution

Single-cell suspension, of either disaggregated tissue, lavage of a body cavity or cultured cells

Protocol

1. With the stock solution of the gradient medium and the chosen diluent, make an aliquot with a density of 1.15 g ml^{-1} (see *Tables 2.3–2.10*).

2. Place the suspension into the tube and underlayer with a volume of the diluted medium sufficient to give a layer about 1–2 cm in depth.

3. Centrifuge in a swinging-bucket rotor for 10–15 min at a speed sufficient to allow all the cells to band at the interface with the medium. Generally, 800–1000 **g** is sufficient, but this will vary a little, depending upon the cell suspension and the types of cells it contains.

4. After centrifugation, all the intact, viable cells should be banded at the sample/medium interface, the dead cells having passed through the medium and pelleted. Harvest viable cells. Most of the cell debris in the cell suspension will remain in the supernatant, being too small to sediment very far at the low speed and short centrifugation time used.

Note

If the presence of stringy aggregates persists then the cell suspension can be treated with a broad range endonuclease to digest the DNA.

Protocol 2.10

Isopycnic separation of rat liver cells using continuous Percoll gradients (Pertoft *et al.*, 1977)

Equipment

Refrigerated centrifuge

Fixed angle rotor

Swing-out rotor with same size tubes as fixed-angle rotor

Centrifuge tubes

Pasteur pipets

Reagents

Percoll

Hepes pH 7.0

60% (w/v) sucrose

Rat liver cell preparation

Protocol

1. Centrifuge 80 ml 10 mM Hepes-buffered Percoll solution in the fixed-angle rotor at 20 000 g for 10 min, generating a continuous gradient of 1.03–1.10 g ml^{-1} Percoll.

2. Layer 15 ml of rat liver cell suspension (2–4 $\times$ 10^{6} cells ml^{-1}) (cf. *Protocol 2.9*) on to the preformed gradient, transfer the tubes to the swing-out rotor and centrifuge at 800 g for 60 min at 4°C.

3. Fractionate gradient by upward displacement using 60% (w/v) sucrose.

4. The cells are localized in three regions of the continuous Percoll gradient. Nonviable cells accumulate on top of the gradient, while phagocytic, nonparenchymal cells (Kupffer cells) band between 1.04 and 1.06 g ml^{-1} and parenchymal cells (hepatocytes) band between 1.07 and 1.09 g ml^{-1}.

5. Count the number of cells in each fraction.

Note

Assay for viability using trypan blue exclusion test, phagocytic activity (by uptake of polystyrene latex particles), and function.

Protocol 2.11

Isolation of hepatocytes by differential pelleting

Equipment

Refrigerated centrifuge with swinging-bucket rotor

Centrifuge tubes

Pasteur pipets

Reagents

Incubation medium

Harvested rat liver cells

Protocol

1. Dilute the harvested cell-band with ice-cold incubation medium in to a volume of 40–60 ml.

2. Place the cell suspension into centrifuge tubes and centrifuge at 50 g for 1 min at 4°C.

3. Decant supernatants carefully (retain if needed for preparation of nonparenchymal cells) and resuspend pellets in same volume as before of ice-cold incubation medium.

4. Repeat centrifugation Step 2.

5. Discard supernatants, resuspend pellets in small volume and examine for purity. If necessary, wash once more.

Note

This procedure should provide a suspension of almost pure hepatocytes. If necessary, this suspension can be processed following *Protocol 2.8*, to remove any cells damaged during the washing steps.

Protocol 2.12

Fractionation of sinusoidal cells (Brouwer *et al.*, 1992)

Equipment

Two-chamber type gradient-mixer

Abbé refractometer

Refrigerated centrifuge with swing-out rotor

Corex 15-ml centrifuge tubes

Pasteur pipets

Reagents

Gey's balanced salt solution (GBSS); 0.14 M NaCl, 5 mM KCl, 0.3 mM MgSO$_4$, 1 mM NaH$_2$PO$_4$, 1.5 mM CaCl$_2$, 3 mM NaHCO$_3$, 0.2 mM KH$_2$PO$_4$, 1 mM MgCl$_2$, 5.5 mM D-glucose, adjusted to pH 7.4 and 275–285 mOsm

28.7% (w/v) Nycodenz in GBSS without NaCl; pH 7.4, 285 mOsm

Nonparenchymal cells

Protocol

Sample preparation

1. Use freshly isolated nonparenchymal cells (2–3 × 10^6 cells) from one rat liver.

2. Wash cells three times by suspension in 15 ml of GBSS and pellet at 300 *g* for 5 min at room temperature. This reduces the risk of cell clumping and removes most of the contaminating parenchymal cell debris.

3. Resuspend the final pellet of cells in 6 ml GBSS.

Gradient preparation and centrifugation

1. Dilute the stock solution of 28.7% (w/v) Nycodenz with GBSS to a concentration of 19.1%. This is the dense solution for preparation of the gradient.

2. Dilute an aliquot of the dense (19.1%) solution with GBSS to obtain a 7.7% (w/v) light solution for the gradient.

3. Prepare a continuous gradient, 7.7–19.1% (w/v) Nycodenz, using the gradient maker.

4. Centrifuge the gradient at 2000 *g* for 30 min at 4°C in a swing-out rotor, using slow acceleration and deceleration. To avoid cell clumping the time of centrifugation should not exceed 45 min.

Analysis of gradients

1. Fractionate the gradient using upward displacement, into fractions of 0.5 ml.

2. Determine the refractive index (RI) of each fraction and calculate the corresponding density using the following equation;

$$\text{Density (g ml}^{-1}) = (\text{RI} \times 3.242) - 3.323. \tag{2.7}$$

3. Determine cell number and viability for each fraction.

4. Determine the distribution of Kupffer, endothelial, and other cells by peroxidase staining.

Protocol 2.13

The isolation and purification of plant protoplasts using OptiPrep gradients

Equipment

Refrigerated centrifuge with swinging-bucket rotor

Centrifuge tubes

9-cm plastic Petri dishes

Nylon mesh, pore size 100 μm

Reagents

Liquid nitrogen

1% sodium hypochlorite/0.01% (v/v) Tween 80

70% ethanol

Distilled water

Plasmolysing solution; 5 mM MES, 1 mM KH_2PO_4, 0.44 M D-sorbitol, 5 mM $CaCl_2$, 2 mM $MgCl_2$, 2 mM $MnCl_2$, 1 mM L-arginine, 1 mM dithiothreitol (DTT), 0.1% (w/v) Polyvinylpyrrolidone-10 (PVP-10), 2 mM glutathione, 2 mM L-ascorbic acid, 0.01% (w/v) trypsin inhibitor soybean S1, 1300 U ml^{-1} catalase. The pH is adjusted to 5.7

Digesting solution; as plasmolysing solution with addition of 2% (w/v) Cellulysin and 0.5% (w/v) macerase

Isolation buffer; as plasmolysing solution without the catalase or trypsin inhibitor

OptiPrep solution; as result of the osmolality measurements taken of the leaf tissue, the osmolality of the OptiPrep is increased to 500 mOsm by addition of 0.6% (w/v) KCl (0.6 g added to 100 ml of OptiPrep)

Seeds of wheat (*Triticum aestivum* L. cv. Mercia) and barley (*Hordeum vulgare* L. cv. Pipkin) sown on Levington potting compost and grown for six days at 25°C with a 16 h photoperiod of 50 μmol m^{-2}s^{-1} in a growth chamber.

Protocol

Determination of leaf osmolality (Sarhan and Cesar, 1988)

1. Powder 3 **g** of leaf tissue in liquid nitrogen, allow to thaw.

2. Centrifuge at 30 000 **g** for 20 min at 4°C.

3. The osmolality of the supernatant is measured using a depression of freezing point osmometer. The osmolality of all incubating solutions is set at 1.8 times that of the tissue.

Protoplast isolation (Sarhan and Cesar, 1988)

1. Remove leaf blades and surface sterilize in 1% sodium hypochlorite/0.01% (v/v) Tween 80 for 5 min.

2. Rinse the tissue three times with distilled water and transfer to 70% (v/v) ethanol for 2 min then wash the tissue a further three times with distilled water. This procedure not only surface sterilizes the tissue but also weakens the cuticle thus aiding protoplast release.

3. Place the leaf tissue in the plasmolysing solution (50 ml g^{-1} tissue) for 30 min at 20°C.

4. Remove the leaves from the solution and cut in to 0.5–1-mm pieces and place in 9-cm Petri plates containing the digesting solution (10 ml g^{-1} tissue).

5. Digest the tissue at 20°C, with shaking at 40 r.p.m. for the first and last 30 min.

6. After digestion, filter the contents of each culture plate, containing 2 g of leaf tissue, through Nylon mesh (pore size 100 μm). Wash off tissue retained by the mesh in isolation buffer, mash it lightly to release more protoplasts, and again filter.

7. Wash the mesh through with the buffer and make up the volume of filtrate from each plate to 30 ml in 50-ml tubes.

Centrifugation

1. Add 7.5 ml of the prepared OptiPrep to each tube to make up a final density of close to 1.07 g ml^{-1} – the density of the diluting medium must be taken into account when calculating the density of the diluted aliquots.

2. Overlayer the mixture with 20 ml of an OptiPrep solution, diluted to about 1.03 g ml^{-1} by mixing 20 ml of the isolation buffer with 2 ml of the prepared OptiPrep.

3. Finally, overlayer 2–3 ml of the isolation buffer on top.

4. Centrifuge at 200 *g* for 4 min in a swinging-bucket rotor at 4°C.

5. After centrifugation, a band of material is found at the top of the medium and in the overlying buffer. There is clear medium from the band down to the 1.03/1.07 g ml^{-1} interface. The 1.07 g ml^{-1} layer contains particulate material and a pellet is found at the bottom of the tube. The band at the top can best be harvested using a plastic Pasteur pipet with the tip cut off to increase the size of the orifice and reduce damage to the protoplasts during harvesting. This band contains over 95% intact protoplasts, with the remainder just showing signs of lysis and loss of chloroplasts. There are an insignificant number of intact protoplasts in the 1.07 g ml^{-1} layer.

Note

The protoplasts are in high concentration and free of any residual enzyme activity, so there is no need to wash the isolated protoplasts, which are harvested in the buffer that contains a small amount of OptiPrep (about 2% Iodixanol) which is not harmful to cells. The practice of washing cells by pelleting and resuspending them several times is very damaging. The method described in this protocol avoids this step.

Protocol 2.14

Isolation of immunologically distinct cell subpopulations using density perturbation methods

Equipment

Refrigerated centrifuge with swinging-bucket rotor

Microcentrifuge

End-over-end mixer

Gradient Master

Sterilin screw cap centrifuge tubes, 12 ml total capacity

Microcentrifuge tubes

Pasteur pipets

Reagents

Either avidin-coated dense polystyrene beads or sheep anti-mouse coated Dynabeads M-450 (Dynal UK)

PBS

Biotinylated affinity-isolated rabbit immunoglobulins to mouse immunoglobulins

0.1% (w/v) bovine serum albumin (BSA) in PBS

Monoclonal mouse antibody to human T cell CD6

OptiPrep solution, 1.32 g ml^{-1}, 260 mOsm

Diluent; 3 mM KCl, 0.3 mM CaEDTA, 5 mM Tricine–NaOH pH 7.2, 0.85% (w/v) NaCl (pH 7, 285 mOsm)

MOLT-4 T cells grown in RPMI 1640 supplemented with 10% fetal calf serum

Protocol

Preparation of beads for labeling cells

1. Wash 3.9 mg of avidin-coated dense polystyrene beads or 3.6 mg Dynabeads M-450 twice in 250 µl PBS and pellet the beads using a microcentrifuge at 18 600 *g* for 15 min at room temperature.

2. Resuspend and incubate 5 × 10^7 avidin-coated dense polystyrene beads with 15 µg biotinylated rabbit anti-mouse immunoglobulins in PBS in a final volume of 125 µl, mix the suspension on an end-over-end mixer at 15 r.p.m. for 45 min at room temperature.

3. Wash the beads twice with 0.1% (w/v) (BSA) in PBS and once with PBS, pellet beads by centrifugation as described in Step 1.

4. Resuspend and incubate the biotinylated rabbit anti-mouse-coated dense polystyrene beads or the Dynabeads M-450 (5×10^7) with 3 µg mouse anti-human CD6 immunoglobulins as described in Step 2, mix for 60 min.

5. Wash the antibody-coated dense beads as described in Step 3.

Bead binding by cells

1. Resuspend 5×10^7 antibody-coated dense beads in 0.1 ml PBS and incubate with viable MOLT-4 T cells (2.5×10^6) in a final volume of 1 ml PBS, in a 1.5-ml microcentrifuge tube. Use a minimum of a 20:1 bead to cell ratio.

2. Mix the suspension on the end-over-end mixer at 15 r.p.m. for 1 h at 25°C.

Fractionation of cells

1. Prepare 1.03 g ml^{-1} and 1.27 g ml^{-1} working OptiPrep solutions as follows.

    (a) To prepare 1.03 g ml^{-1} solution dilute stock OptiPrep with diluent, 1 to 11 parts respectively.

    (b) To prepare 1.27 g ml^{-1} solution dilute stock OptiPrep with diluent, 5 to 1 parts respectively.

2. By gentle inversion of Sterilin tube, mix 1 ml labeled cell suspension with 2.5 ml 1.03 g ml^{-1} OptiPrep and 1.5 ml diluent to obtain 1.02 g ml^{-1} initial solution.

3. Underlayer with 5 ml 1.27 g ml^{-1} OptiPrep.

4. Prepare an isotonic continuous 1.02–1.27 g ml^{-1} OptiPrep gradient (osmolality range 290–310 mOsm) by rotation using a Gradient master (80°, 20 r.p.m., 2 min).

5. Centrifuge the gradient at 220 g_{max} for 90 min at 20°C, for this use a bench-top centrifuge without applying the brake.

6. Recover cells that have not bound beads from the top of the gradient. Cells associated with antibody-coated dense beads are found in denser regions of the gradient.

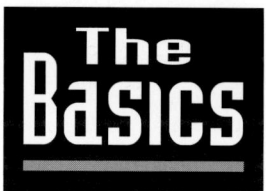

Chapter 3

Centrifugal elutriation

1. Introduction

In centrifugal elutriation, cells are separated according to their rate of sedimentation in a gravitational field where the liquid containing the cells is made to flow against the gravitational force. The liquid used is of uniform density and flows toward the center of rotation through a conical shaped chamber, the apex of which points away from the center of rotation. Cells are thus subjected to two opposing forces within the separation chamber, a centrifugal force generated by the spinning rotor and the centripetal flow of the fluid (*Figures 3.1* and *3.2*). Each cell migrates to a zone in the chamber where the two forces acting on them are at equilibrium. The position of each cell is determined mainly by its size, however, shape and density also have an effect. Since a uniform, low-density medium is used, sedimentation rate is proportional to cell size. Cells of different size tend to accumulate in discrete sections of the chamber. Smaller cells accumulate nearer the center of rotation, larger cells further from the center. As the geometry of the chamber produces a gradient of flow rates from one end to the other, cells with a wide range of different sedimentation rates can be held in suspension at one time. No pelleting occurs and the fractions can be eluted by increasing the flow rate of the liquid or decreasing the centrifugal force.

Centrifugal elutriation is both a rapid and noninvasive method for the preparation of specific subpopulations of cells from mixed cell types. First described by Lindberg (1932), and later refined by Lindahl (1948), this

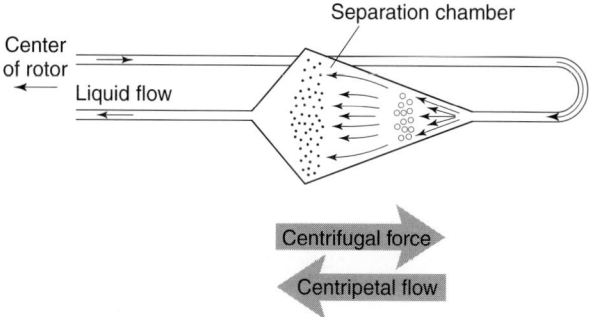

Figure 3.1

Schematic showing separation by centrifugal elutriation from Freshney, R.I. (1994) Culture of Animal Cells, *3rd edn, with permission from John Wiley & Sons Ltd.*

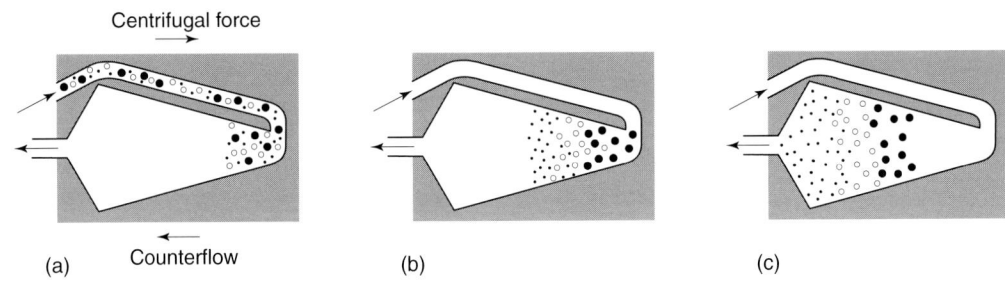

Figure 3.2

Cross-sectional diagrams of a standard separation chamber during cell separation. Centrifugal force is opposed by a counterflow of elutriation buffer. (a) A mixed cell population is loaded into the chamber; (b) cell subpopulations begin to separate out as the buffer flow rate is increased; (c) as the flow rate is again increased, the smallest cells begin to elute from the chamber.

technique, originally termed 'counterstreaming centrifugation', has since become widely used for the separation of cells from an extremely diverse range of sources.

2.   Principles

The basis for separating cells of varying diameters and densities within a given medium is best described by Stokes' law (cf. Chapter 2):

$$v_s = \frac{2}{9} \times \frac{r^2(\rho_p - \rho_m)g}{\mu} \qquad (3.1)$$

where v_s=velocity of sedimentation, r=radius of particle, ρ_p=density of particle, ρ_m=density of medium, μ=viscosity of medium, and g=gravitational or centrifugal force.

The concept of centrifugal elutriation was devised by Lindberg (1932). He showed that cell fractions could be resolved by 'washing' a cell suspension whilst it was undergoing centrifugation. Lindberg devised a conical chamber that was aligned in the centrifuge such that cells or other particles were subjected to opposing forces; the centrifugal force generated by the spinning of the rotor and the fluid counterflow in the opposite (centripetal) direction. The flow rate of the suspending medium through the chamber was such that it was too high to permit the cells to sediment, but was also too low to wash the cells out of the chamber. The principle of the original 'counterstreaming centrifuge' and its modern day counterparts is essentially the same. Whilst there may be other manufacturers of elutriation chambers and centrifuges, by far the most widely available and used are those by Beckman.

The design of the separation chamber is critical to its performance. The geometry of the chambers is such that there is an increasing cross-sectional area, and in turn, a decreasing velocity of flow of the suspension medium, toward the center of the rotor (*Figures 3.1* and *3.2*). The cells or particles within the chamber are subjected to two opposing forces; the centrifugal field generated by the spinning rotor, and the viscous drag of the elutriation buffer or medium flowing at a particular rate (v_f) in the opposite direction. After loading the chamber with cells, each cell equilibrates at a position within the chamber where its sedimentation velocity (v_s) is equal to v_f. This is defined by Equation 3.2:

$$v_s = v_f = \frac{F}{A} = \frac{d^2(\rho_p - \rho_m)(\omega^2 r)}{18\mu} \qquad (3.2)$$

where F=flow rate of the elutriation buffer or medium (ml min^{-1}), A=cross-sectional area (cm^2), d=particle diameter (μm), and $\omega^2 r$=angular velocity of the rotor.

Where the density of a cell type is known, at a given rotor speed the approximate elutriation flow rate at which the cell will remain in the chamber can be determined.

As the cross-sectional area of the chamber changes, a flow rate gradient is generated within the chamber and this enables mixtures of cells with a large range of sedimentation velocities to be held in suspension. By increasing the flow rate of the buffer (or by reducing the rotor speed) in small incremental steps, different subpopulations of relatively homogeneous cell size can be eluted from the chamber. Each successive fraction will contain cells that are larger or denser than those of the previous fraction. Therefore, accurate and precise fractionation of cells with extremely small differences in size and/or density can be achieved.

3.   Equipment

The equipment required for centrifugal elutriation comprises a large capacity slow/medium speed centrifuge with a modified lid, a separation chamber and rotor assembly, a high-performance variable flow rate pump, and a stroboscope assembly.

3.1   Centrifuge

Unlike the separation of cells by sedimentation methods (Chapter 2), only a limited number of centrifuges are suitable for centrifugal elutriation. A centrifuge with a precise, linear, and highly reproducible rotor speed is essential, as the rotor speed must be finely controlled. Any disturbance in the rotor speed experienced during the run and elution will result in disturbance of the equilibrium within the separation chamber and consequently mixing of cell populations.

Centrifuges can be fitted with a stroboscope in the base of the bowl and an observation port in the centrifuge lid to allow visualization of cell elutriation within the chamber. A fixed image of the revolving chamber is obtained by synchronizing the stroboscope flash rate with the rotor speed. Banding of cells in the chamber can be seen through the window enabling the operator to control the elution of cells from the chamber.

3.2   Separation chamber and rotor assembly

Based on the separations obtained by Lindahl and colleagues, Beckman produced a series of elutriator rotors from the mid-1960s resulting in the versions currently available, the JE-6B and JE-5.0. The JE-6B system comprises a single separation chamber with a volume of approximately 5 ml and a bypass chamber on the opposite side of the rotor. The chamber is made of transparent synthetic material, which allows illumination by a stroboscopic lamp and visualization during the elutriation run via an observation port in the lid of the centrifuge (*Figure 3.3*). The JE-5.0 system incorporates interchangeable small and large standard chambers as well as the Sanderson chamber (described below). Although this system can be used with two separation chambers in series, it is more usual to use a single chamber and counterbalance.

The three separation chambers used routinely in the aforementioned systems are the standard and Sanderson chambers of the JE-6B and JE-5.0 systems, and the large standard chamber which can only be used in the JE-5.0 rotor assembly. The designs of the small and large standard chambers are essentially the same, and differ only in their volumes. The larger chamber is used when the number of cells to be separated is increased. A key difference between the standard and Sanderson chamber, is that in the latter, the walls of the chamber diverge rapidly at a point of entry whilst the walls of the upper section are almost parallel (*Figure 3.4*). This results in a wider separation of cells in the upper section and thus the separation of cells with only very small differences in their physical characteristics.

3.3 Pump

An even, consistent and nonpulsatile flow of buffer through the separation chamber is essential. Fluctuations in the flow rate, however minor, will adversely influence the equilibrium within the chamber during the run and reduce the efficiency, quality, and reproducibility of the separation. To minimize any variation in flow rate, the pump should be of high quality and be calibrated before each separation and tubing checked for wear.

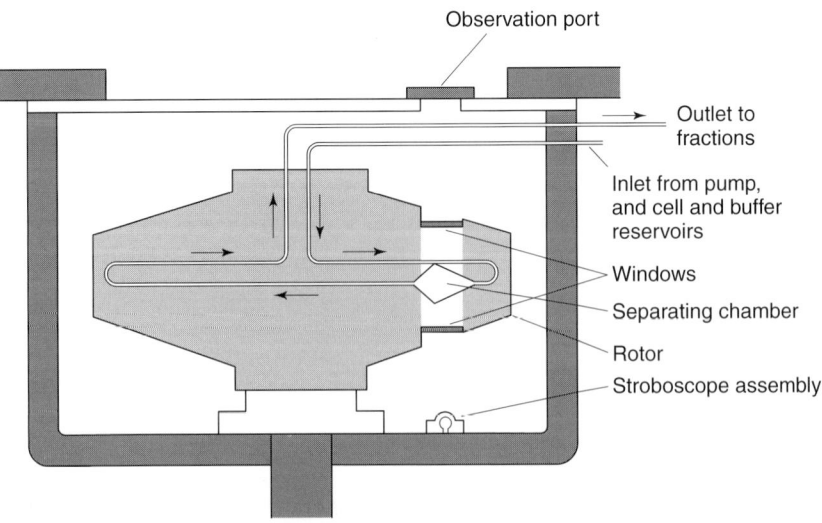

Figure 3.3

Diagram showing a centrifugal elutriator rotor (Beckman JE-6B).

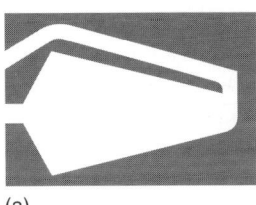

(a)

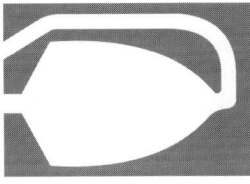

(b)

Figure 3.4

Schematic showing a comparison of the standard (a) and the Sanderson (b) separation chambers.

Protocol 3.1 describes the basic procedure used when setting-up a centrifugal elutriation system.

4.   Conditions affecting separation

A crucial step in centrifugal elutriation is the preparation of a completely homogeneous single cell suspension. This is relatively easy for cell preparations from some tissues where following disaggregation, repeat-pipeting of the loading suspension through a Pasteur pipet may suffice. However, for adherent cell lines growing in monolayers it is essential to disaggregate both fully and carefully. For this purpose, in addition to gentle trypsin treatment, the addition of DNase to degrade any free DNA released from lysed cells is recommended to prevent cell clumping. This can also be included in the loading suspension or elutriation buffer. Blood cells have the advantage of occurring naturally as nonadherent cells and lend themselves particularly well to the preparation of enriched fractions by centrifugal elutriation.

The choice of elutriation buffer or medium is dependent upon the cell type to be separated. Serum-containing culture medium may also be used but this may prove expensive as fractions are collected in volumes of 80–100 ml using the small volume chambers and up to 1000 ml if the large standard chamber is used. Supplementing the elutriation buffer with agents such as DNase I, EDTA (a divalent cation chelator), hydroxymethyl-amino methane 2-(N-morpholine)propane sulfonic acid (MOPS) (Lauf and Bauer, 1987), 4-(2-hydroxyethyl)-1-piperazine ethanesulfonic acid (PIPES) or polyvinylpyrrolidone (PVP) (Watkins *et al.*, 1992) is used to reduce any cell clumping.

The number and density of cells that can be loaded into a chamber at any one time depends on the type of chamber and also to some extent on the size range of the cells. The standard and Sanderson chambers have capacity for up to 10^9 cells while the large standard chamber can accommodate up to 10^{10} cells. The maximum number of cells per chamber is limited by the ability of cells of different sizes to form discrete bands in the chamber. Overloading the chamber may encourage clumping of the cells or adversely affect the flow equilibrium. When many cells are present the adjacent bands may overlap. The precise numbers depend on the number of bands that form and on the size of cells; larger cells will tend to form broader bands. When smaller numbers of cells are used, problems can sometimes occur even when these numbers are within the minimum range of the chamber. Turbulence in the chamber can occur as the buffer flows through with small cell numbers. Any such turbulence is 'buffered' with larger cell numbers by the cell bulk. When turbulence does occur resolution is reduced since discrete bands of cells cannot form. One way of avoiding turbulence with small numbers of cells is to increase the viscosity of the elutriation buffer by inclusion of high molecular weight molecules as Ficoll, dextran or BSA in the fluid. A reduction in cell recovery can also occur with low cell numbers, since there is a lower limit to the number of cells which should be loaded: 2×10^7 in the small standard, 2×10^6 in the Sanderson, and 2×10^8 in the large standard.

The temperature of the fluid (elutriation buffer) used in elutriator separations is a major factor in obtaining cell separations. The optimum temperature for any particular separation is dependent on the type of cells. Most work with isolated cells is conducted at 4°C and many successful elutriator separations have been achieved at this temperature. If no published conditions are available for a particular cell type to be separated, it is advisable to conduct several elutriator separations at different temperatures to obtain the optimum conditions to achieve the separation and recovery required. To ensure good reproducibility, elutriation at a constant temperature is important. While most cells remain stable for longer at lower temperatures and at low population densities, cell membranes are less fluid at such temperatures and are therefore more susceptible to shear forces, which might result in disruption of the plasma membrane and cell damage. Yet, at higher temperatures, cells are more prone to clumping. It is important to ensure that the chosen temperature is maintained throughout the procedure, as it is vital that the viscosity of the medium does not fluctuate and disturb the equilibrium within the chamber. However, it is important to note that where cells with large size differences are being separated, small fluctuations in temperature will not greatly affect separation. The control of temperature is more important where the size differences are small, that is, at the limits of the resolving power of the apparatus.

After each run it is essential to remove all cellular, proteinaceous and particulate material from the system. This can be achieved by several means including soaking the separation chamber for several hours in KOH and then thoroughly rinsing in distilled water. Once assembled in the rotor, the chamber and the entire flow system should be flushed with approximately 200–300 ml of distilled water followed by 200 ml of elutriation buffer. Alternatively, the system is flushed with distilled water, followed by a weak solution of a neutral detergent such as Tween 80, and finally with distilled water. If required the whole elutriator system can be sterilized by passing 500 ml of 70% ethanol or 500 ml hydrogen peroxide through the system. The protocol used should be checked against the equipment specifications to ensure compatibility to avoid corrosion, *et cetera*.

5.   Applications of centrifugal elutriation

With the development of the sophisticated instrumentation necessary, the applications to which centrifugal elutriation has been applied have increased enormously. This is not surprising when the whole run may take only 30 min depending on the cell type, on each run 10^8 cells may be separated, and fractionation may be repeated as often as necessary. The technique is rapid and cell yield is high. Examples of separation by centrifugal elutriation include the separation of blood cells into purified populations including platelets, erythrocytes, lymphocytes and monocytes; separation of cells from solid tissues and tumors; growth synchronization of proliferating cell lines, and separation of subpopulations of a single cell type. The technique has also been used in the purification of yeast, bacterial and plant cells. Detailed below are selected examples that illustrate the variety of different conditions that can be used to achieve cell separation.

5.1 Synchronized cells

As proliferating cells progress through successive phases of the growth cycle, namely G_1, S-phase, and G_2, they increase in size. Following mitosis (M), two smaller daughter cells are produced. The daughter cells enter a further cycle commencing again with G_1. This size differential between cells at different stages of the cell cycle is used as the basis for separation of relatively large yields of growth synchronous cells by centrifugal elutriation. The degree of success by elutriation compares favorably with alternative methods of synchronizing cells which involve the use of reagents to reversibly block cells at various stages of the cycle, or require other means of physical separation (Lloyd *et al.*, 1982). However, centrifugal elutriation yields much higher numbers of cells and separation is complete in less than 50 min. Where only one selected fraction is desired the time is further reduced. Other means of synchronizing cells can take much longer, even as much as 2–3 days. An example for the preparation of synchronized mouse L-P59 fibroblasts is described in *Protocol 3.2*. Various examples of cell types separated into growth synchronous populations by elutriation are summarized in *Table 3.1*. In prokaryotes, centrifugal elutriation has been used for studies of cell cycle-specific gene expression. It has been used in lower eukaryotes, for example, to separate yeast cells (Aves *et al.*, 1985), for studies in understanding the genes regulating the control of the cell cycle, and even with plant cells (Pomponi and Cucci, 1989).

5.2 Blood cells

Blood cells have the advantage of occurring naturally as nonadherent cells (in suspension) and so lend themselves particularly well to the preparation of enriched fractions by centrifugal elutriation. Elutriation exploits both size and density differentials existent between the various cell types which comprise blood. The platelets are the smallest cells present in blood and will elute first. Erythrocytes are the largest and are usually separated by a process of elimination, by eluting the smaller cells out of the chamber thereby leaving the erythrocyte fraction. In addition, erythrocytes are not a uniform size, they become smaller and denser as they mature, and therefore can be separated into different age groups (Jansen *et al.*, 1986). For the separation of granulocyte, lymphocyte, leukocyte and monocyte preparations, it is usual to start with an initial step prior to elutriation. This might be lysis of red cells, density gradient centrifugation or some other method. A variety of cell separations from blood using centrifugal elutriation are exemplified in *Table 3.2*.

5.3 Liver cells

Several different cell types comprise the liver. These include the hepatocytes or parenchymal cells, Kupffer cells, fat-storing cells, sinusoidal epithelial cells and biliary epithelial cells. The hepatocytes or parenchymal cells make up the largest proportion of the total cell population (approximately 70%). Centrifugal elutriation is frequently used to isolate the various cell populations that constitute this tissue as exemplified in *Table 3.3*. In addition, centrifugal elutriation has been used with hepatocyte preparations to fractionate subpopulations of single cells and to purify hepatocyte couplets which

Table 3.1. Selected examples of cell types separated into growth synchronous populations by centrifugal elutriation

Cell type	Elutriation buffer	Loading conditions			Temp (°C)	Comments	Ref.
		Cell number	Speed (r.p.m.)	Flow (ml min⁻¹)			
Human							
Cervical carcinoma HeLa	PBS, 0.3 mM EDTA, 1% (v/v) FCS, 0.1% (w/v) glucose	8×10^{10}	1550	65	4	Waste 500 ml, then collect 11 fractions at 75–190 ml min⁻¹	Draetta and Beach (1988); Buchkovich et al. (1989)
Erythropoietic cells		10^{10}	3000	65		Fractions collected at 75–300 ml min⁻¹	Virshup et al. (1989)
Mouse							
Erythroleukemia cells	DMEM, 7.5 (v/v) FCS	10^{9}	2000	15	22	Waste initially. Collect cells at 15–35 ml min⁻¹	Braunstein et al. (1982)
Fibroblasts 3T3	DMEM, 10% (v/v) FCS	3×10^{8}	2000	10.2	5	Waste at 15 ml min⁻¹ Collect at 20 ml min⁻¹	Mitchell and Tupper (1977)
L-P59 fibroblasts	McCoys 5A medium, 5% (v/v) FCS, 5 nM 2-naphthol-6,8-disulfonic acid	3×10^{7}	1525	9	4	Collected 12 fractions at 9–25.6 ml min⁻¹	Meistrich et al. (1977)
Fibrosarcoma	McCoys 5A medium 5% (v/v) FCS, 5 nM 2-naphthol-6,8-disulfonic acid	2×10^{8}	1210	7.4	4	Collected 12 fractions at 7.4–31.4 ml min⁻¹	Suzuki et al. (1977)
Other							
Schizosaccharomyces pombe		3×10^{10}	2100	100	25	Waste to 120 ml min⁻¹. Collect at 120, 130, 140 ml min⁻¹	Aves et al. (1985)
Yeast	Culture medium pH 5.4, 2% (w/v) glucose, 0.5% (w/v) $(NH_4)_2SO_4$, 4.7 g l⁻¹ NaCl	10^{10}	2750	10	4	Waste for 30 min. Collect 10–14 ml	Woldringh et al. (1993)

Table 3.2. Selected protocols for the separation of blood cells using centrifugal elutriation

Cell type	Elutriation buffer	Loading conditions				Comments	Ref.
		Cell number	Speed (r.p.m.)	Flow (ml min⁻¹)	Temp (°C)		
Platelets	105.5 mM NaCl, 128 mM Na$_2$HPO$_4$, 2.8 mM KH$_2$PO$_4$, 15% (w/v) fatty acid-free BSA	5 ml of 5–9 × 10^9	4000	1	22	Waste to 2 ml min⁻¹, then collect cells at 4, 6, 8 and 10 ml min⁻¹	Van Prooijen et al. (1989)
Monocytes	pH 7.2 PBS, 5% (w/v) dextrose, 1–2% (v/v) horse serum albumin	1 × 10^9	2080	8		Run at 11 ml min⁻¹ for 60 min to remove lymphocytes. Collect remainder monocytes	Clouse et al. (1989)
Human monocytes	Lymphocyte separation medium (LSM)		2000			Lymphocyte-rich (90%) at 12–16 ml min⁻¹. Monocyte rich (>90%) at 17–20 ml min⁻¹	Maeda et al. (1991)
Human monocytes and lymphocytes	PBS 5% FCS, 0.01% EDTA	1.5–3.75 × 10^8	1950	10	18	Run 10 ml min⁻¹ followed by 0.5 ml min⁻¹ increments every 8 min up to 14 ml min⁻¹. Collect cells in 13 fractions of 50 ml each	Yasaka et al. (1981)
Lymphocytes Lymphocytes	Seligmann's buffer	1.5 × 10^9 10^7–10^8	3000 3000	12 11	10 4	Collect cells at 18 and 28 ml min⁻¹. Collect successive fractions with 15, 17, 19 and 21% BSA solutions	Zucali et al. (1987) Griffith (1978)
Leukocytes	Krebs Ringer phosphate buffer pH 7.6, 0.15 mM glucose, 1% (w/v) BSA		2000	7.8	15	Collect lymphocytes at 10–12.5 ml min⁻¹, monocytes 14–17.5 ml min⁻¹, and remainder 19 ml min⁻¹	Fogelman et al. (1977)
Bovine lymphocytes	HBSS	6 × 10^8	2430	10		Collect 9 fractions at 16–81 ml min⁻¹	Raghunathan et al. (1982)
Human granulocytes	pH 7.45, 150 mM NaCl, 10 mM HEPES, 5 mM KCl, 0.1% (w/v) EDTA, 2% (w/v) heat inactivated FCS	2 × 10^8	2000	10	15	Slow increase to 14.5 ml min⁻¹. Run 10 min. Stop. Centrifuge and collect chamber contents	Tolley et al. (1987)

contd.

Table 3.2. contd.

Cell type	Elutriation buffer	Loading conditions				Comments	Ref.
		Cell number	Speed (r.p.m.)	Flow (ml min⁻¹)	Temp (°C)		
Human basophils	25 mM Pipes, 110 mM NaCl, 5 mM KCl, 0.1% (w/v) glucose, 0.25% BSA		2600	20		Reduce speed to 2500 r.p.m. and waste. Reduce speed to 2300 r.p.m. and collect cells	Warner and MacGlashan (1989)
Human megakaryocytes	HBSS, 3.5% (v/v) BSA, 3.8% Na citrate, 2 mM theophyline, 1 mM adenosine	5×10^8	1000	7		Run to waste for at least 150 ml. Run at 800 r.p.m. and 15 ml min⁻¹. Waste 200 ml. Collect remaining cells	Gewirtz and Shen (1990)
Rat pituitary cell	Ca- and Mg-free Dulbecco's balanced salt solution pH 7.4, 1% (w/v) BSA, 6 g l⁻¹ HEPES, 10 mg l⁻¹ gentamycin	$5{-}15 \times 10^6$ (in DNase)	1920	8	6-8	Collect at 15 ml min⁻¹ (small), 25 ml min⁻¹ (medium), 35 ml min⁻¹ (large)	Childs et al. (1992)
Rat lung cells	HBSS, 1000 U ml⁻¹ DNase I	$5{-}6 \times 10^8$	2500	8.5		Reduce spin speed to 2200 r.p.m., waste 100 ml. Collect 10-18 ml min⁻¹. 1200 r.p.m. collect 18 ml min⁻¹	Lacy et al. (1992)
Porcine neutrophils	PBS, 0.2% (w/v) gelatin, 0.1% (w/v) glucose		2370	4	25	Waste to 6 ml min⁻¹, then collect cells in 2 ml min⁻¹ increments to 22 ml min⁻¹	
Ovine reticulocytes	145 mM NaNO₃, 5 mM glucose, 10mM Tris-MOPS pH 7.4	25% (v/v) suspension	3000	5	5	Collect at 9–24 ml min⁻¹	Lauf and Bauer (1987)

Table 3.3. Selected protocols for the separation of specific liver cells from mixed populations using centrifugal elutriation

Cell type	Elutriation buffer	Loading conditions				Comments	Ref.
		Cell number	Speed (r.p.m.)	Flow (ml min⁻¹)	Temp (°C)		
Murine Kupffer cells	GBSS, 0.05% (v/v) FCS		2500	21	4	Collect 200 ml to waste. Collect cells at 40 ml min⁻¹	Janousek et al. (1993)
Rat liver cells	Leibowitz-15 medium, 0.001% (w/v) DNase I, 0.2% (w/v) Protease XIV		2500	12		Sinusoidal epithelial cells collected at 12–18 ml min⁻¹. Kupffer cells collected at 30–44 ml min⁻¹	McCloskey et al. (1992)
Rat hepatocytes	Krebs–Henseleit pH 7.4, 20 mM PIPES, 5 mM glucose, 1% (w/v) PVP, 50 mg ml⁻¹ DNase I	1.25×10^8	1700	19	8	Waste to 27 ml min⁻¹. Collect at 33 ml min⁻¹, then at 50 ml min⁻¹, finally at 60 ml min⁻¹	Watkins et al. (1992)
Rat Kupffer and endothelial cells	GBSS		2500	20		Collect 250 ml at 20 ml min⁻¹. Increase to 42 ml min⁻¹ and collect 150 ml for 3–4 min	Knook and Sleyster (1976); Zahlten et al. (1978)
Rat Kupffer cells	GBSS, 0.001% (w/v) DNase, 0.2% (w/v) pronase		875 **g**	23		Waste to 29 ml min⁻¹. Collect small cells at 45 ml min⁻¹. Reduce rotor to 1 **g** and collect remainder	Jaeschke et al. (1992)
Rat fat-storing cells	HBSS		3250	10		Collect cells at 16–18 ml min⁻¹	Sakamoto et al. (1993)

are used in bile synthesis and secretion studies (*Protocol 3.3*). Cell purity is verified by morphological analysis using phase-contrast microscopy or by immunochemical or histochemical markers of specific cell types.

6.   Advantages and disadvantages

Centrifugal elutriation offers several advantages over other established methods of cell separation and purification. However, as with any specialized technique there are also a number of disadvantages. These are listed below.

Advantages:

- choice of medium used for elutriation is adaptable – cells that are particularly sensitive can be maintained throughout elutriation in the optimal medium even serum-containing culture medium;
- separations can be performed at any required temperature;
- up to 10^{10} cells can be accommodated in a single run – this exceeds by far the number of cells that can be conveniently run on density gradients or other techniques;
- high viability is maintained throughout elutriation runs;
- improved viability of cell preparations – dead and dying cells are generally of much lower density than the viable cells;
- yields of more than 90% of those cells loaded can be obtained;
- sterility can also be maintained during the procedure;
- rapid technique – separation of a loaded cell population can be complete in as little as 15–20 min.

Disadvantages:

- sophisticated and specialized equipment is fairly expensive and a considerable amount of experience is required before effective separations may be made;
- crucial to load a high quality single cell suspension;
- although cells growing as adherent monolayers can be elutriated, it is important to disaggregate them as efficiently as possible to yield a homogeneous cell suspension, a task easier to achieve with some cell lines than others.

References

Aves, S.J., Durkacz, B.W., Carr, A. and Nurse, P. (1985). Cloning, sequencing and transcriptional control of the *Schizosaccharomyces pombe* cdc 'start' gene. *EMBO J.* **4**: 457–463.

Braunstein, J.D., Schulze, D., Delguidice, T. Furst, A. and Schildkraut, C.L. (1982) The temporal order of replication of murine immunoglobulin heavy-chain constant region sequences corresponds to their linear order in the genome. *Nucl. Acid Res.* **10**: 6887–6902.

Buchkovich, K., Duffy, L.A. and Harlow, E. (1989) The retinoblastoma protein is phosphorylated during specific phases of the cell cycle. *Cell* **58**: 1097–1105.

Childs, G.V., Unabia, D. and Lloyd, J. (1992) Recruitment and maturation of small subsets of luteinizing hormone gonadotropes during the estrous cycle. *Endocrinology* **130**: 335–344.

Clouse, K.A., Powell, D., Washington, I. *et al.* (1989) Monokine regulation of HIV-1 expression in a chronically infected human T cell clone. *J. Immunol.* **142**: 431–438.

Draetta, G. and Beach, D. (1988) Activation of cdc-2 protein kinase during mitosis in human cells. *Cell* **54**: 17–26.

Fogelman, A.M., Seager, J., Edwards, P.A., Hokom, M. and Popják, G. (1977) Cholesterol biosynthesis in human lymphocytes, monocytes, and granulocytes. *Biochem. Biophys. Res. Commun.* **76**: 167–173.

Freshney, R.I. (1994) *Culture of Animal Cells,* 3rd Edn. Wiley, Chichester.

Gewirtz, A.M. and Shen, Y.M. (1990) Effect of phorbol myristate acetate on c-myc, beta-actin, and Fv gene expression in morphologically recognizable human megakaryocytes. *Exp. Hematol.* **18**: 945–952.

Griffith, O.M. (1978) Separation of T and B cells from human peripheral blood by centrifugal elutriation. *Anal. Biochem.* **87**: 97–107.

Jaeschke, H., Bautista, A.P., Spolarics, Z. and Spitzer, J.J. (1992) Superoxide generation by neutrophils and Kupffer cells during *in vivo* reperfusion after hepatic ischemia in rats. *J. Leuk. Biol.* **52**: 377–382.

Janousek, J., Strmen, E. and Gervais, F. (1993) Purification of murine Kupffer cells by centrifugal elutriation. *J. Immunol. Methods* **164**: 109–117.

Jansen, G., Hepkema, B.G., Van der Vegt, S.G.L. and Stahl, J.E.G. (1986) Glycolytic activity in human red cell populations separated by a combination of density and counterflow centrifugation. *Scand. J. Hematol.* **37**: 189–195.

Knook, D.L. and Sleyster, E.Ch. (1976) Separation of Kupffer and endothelial cells of the rat liver by centrifugal elutriation. *Exp. Cell Res.* **99**: 444–449.

Lacy, S.A., Mangum, J.B. and Everitt, J.I. (1992) Cytochrome P-450 and glutathione-associated enzyme activities in freshly isolated enriched lung cell fractions from beta-naphthoflavone-treated male F344 rats. *Toxicology* **73**: 147–160.

Lauf, P.K. and Bauer, J. (1987) Direct evidence for chloride-dependent volume reduction in macrocytic sheep reticulocytes. *Biochem. Biophys. Res. Commun.* **144**: 849–855.

Lindahl, P.E. (1948) *Nature* **161**: 648.

Lindberg, C.A. (1932) *Science* **75**: 415.

Lloyd, D., Poole, R.K. and Edwards, S.W. (eds) (1982) In *The Cell Division Cycle: Temporal Organisation and Control of Cellular Growth and Reproduction.* Academic Press, London, pp. 44–93.

Maeda, K., Sone, S., Ohmoto, Y. and Ogura, T. (1991) A novel differentiation antigen on human monocytes that is specifically induced by granulocyte-macrophage colony-stimulating factor or IL-3. *J. Immunol.* **146**: 3779–3784.

McCloskey, T.W., Todaro, J.A. and Laskin, D.L. (1992) Lipopolysaccharide treatment of rats alters antigen expression and oxidative metabolism in hepatic macrophages. *Hepatology* **16**: 191–203.

Meistrich, M.L., Meyn, R.E. and Barlogie, B. (1977) Synchronisation of mouse L-P59 cells by centrifugal elutriation separation. *Exp. Cell Res.* **105**: 169–177.

Mitchell, B.F. and Tupper, J.T. (1977) Synchonization of mouse 3T3 and SV40 3T3 cell by way of centrifugal elutriation. *Exp. Cell Res.* **106**: 351–355.

Pomponi, S.A. and Cucci, T.I. (1989) Separation and concentration of phytoplankton populations using centrifugal elutriation. *Cytometry* **10**: 580–586.

Raghunathan, R., Wuest, C., Faust, J., Hwang, S. and Miller, M.E. (1982) Isolation of ovine lymphocytes, granulocytes and monocytes by counterflow centrifugal elutriation. *Am. J. Vet. Res.* **43**: 1467–1470.

Sakamoto, M., Ueno, T., Kin, M. *et al.* (1993) Synchronisation of mouse L-P59 cells by centrifugal elutriation. *Hepatology* **18**: 978–983.

Suzuki, N., Frapart, M., Grdina, D.J., Meistrich, M.L. and Withers, H.R. (1977) Cell cycle dependency of metastatic lung colony formation. *Cancer Res.* **37**: 3690–3693.

Tolley, J.O., Omann, G.M. and Jesaitis, A.J. (1987) A high yield, high purity elutriation method for preparing human granulocytes demonstrating enhanced experimental lifetimes. *J. Leuk. Biol.* **42**: 43–50.

Van Prooijen, H.C., Van Heugten, J.G., Riemens, M.I. and Akkerman, J.W.N. (1989) Differences in the susceptibility of platelets to freezing damage in relation to size. *Transfusion* **29**: 539–543.

Virshup, D.M., Kauffman, M.G. and Kelly, T.J. (1989) Activation of SV40 DNA replication *in vitro* by cellular protein phosphatase 2A. *EMBO J.* **8**: 3891–3898.

Warner, J.A. and MacGlashan, D.W. (1989) Protein kinase C (PKC) changes in human basophils. *J. Immunol.* **142**: 1669–1677.

Watkins, J.B., Thierau, D. and Schwarz, L.R. (1992) Biotransformation in carcinogen-induced diploid and polyploid hepatocytes separated by centrifugal elutriation. *Cancer Res.* **52**: 1149–1154.

Wilton, J.C., Williams, D.E., Strain, A.J., Parslow, R.A., Chipman, J.K. and Coleman, R. (1991) Purification of hepatocyte couplets by centrifugal elutriation. *Hepatology* **14**: 180–183.

Woldringh, C.L., Huls, P.G. and Vischer, N.O. (1993) Volume growth of daughter and parent cells during the cell cycle of *Saccharomyces cerevisiae* a/α as determined by image cytometry. *J. Bacteriol.* **175**: 3174–3181.

Yasaka, T., Mantich, N.M., Boxer, L.A. and Baehner, R.L. (1981) Functions of human monocyte and lymphocyte subsets obtained by countercurrent centrifugal elutriation. *J. Immunol.* **127**: 1515–1518.

Zahlten, R.N., Hagler, H.W., Nejtek, M.E. and Day, C.J. (1978) Morphological characterization of Kupffer and endothelial cells of rat liver isolated by counterflow elutriation. *Gastroenterology* **75**: 80–87.

Zucali, J.R., Elfenbein, G.J., Barth, K.C. and Dinarello, C.A. (1987) Effects of human IL-1 and human necrosis factor on human T lymphocyte colony formation. *J. Clin. Invest.* **80**: 772–777.

Protocol 3.1

Standard procedure for cell separation by centrifugal elutriation

Equipment

Centrifuge rotor

20-ml syringe

Collection/centrifuge tubes

Reagents

Elutriation buffer

70% (v/v) ethanol or 6% (v/v) hydrogen peroxide

Cell suspension

Protocol

1. Before assembly of the rotor, ensure that the bearings are clean and run smoothly and that the O-rings are in good condition.

2. If maintenance of sterility is required, flush the system through with 70% (v/v) ethanol (or 6% (v/v) hydrogen peroxide) for 15 min.

3. Thereafter flush through with 500 ml of sterile distilled water.

4. Wash the system through with the elutriation buffer ensuring that the first 150–200 ml runs to waste.

5. Purge the whole system of air.

6. Set the rotor speed, temperature, and pump to the loading rate. Check calibration of the pump flow rate at this point.

7. To load sample fill a 20-ml syringe with the concentrated cell suspension ensuring that there are no air bubbles. Carefully inject the cell suspension into the loading chamber via the injection valve so that the cell suspension settles at the bottom of the loading chamber.

8. Invert the loading chamber and to allow the sample to flow into the separation chamber. The cell suspension can be seen to enter the separation chamber by way of the stroboscope-illuminated viewing port and should form a loose pellet at the bottom of the chamber.

9. After a short equilibration period, increase the flow rate at selected increments and collect 100 ml (small standard and Sanderson chamber) or 800 ml (large standard chamber) eluates, although volumes can be adapted to suit specific requirements.

10. Harvest the cells by centrifugation, resuspend in desired volume and analyze as appropriate.

Notes

A light application of silicone grease to O-rings, *et cetera*, will ensure that the joints will remain water-tight.

To purge system of air: (a) remove any air bubbles in the separation chamber by running the rotor up to speed and down again; (b) check for leaks inside the centrifuge bowl at this stage; (c) if leakage has occurred, regrease the O-rings and joints; (d) release bubbles trapped in taps or tubing connectors by pinching off the tubing briefly and releasing after the pressure has increased slightly; and (e) remove air pockets present in the pressure gauge by inverting the gauge.

Inevitably a proportion of the loading suspension will sediment below the outlet needle of the loading chamber, and it is therefore necessary to gently shake the tube a number of times to ensure that all the cells are loaded. It is vital that no air bubbles are allowed to enter the rotor.

Protocol 3.2

Separation of growth synchronous cells

Equipment

Centrifuge rotor

Phase-contrast microscope

Pasteur pipets

Collection/centrifuge tubes

Reagents

Elutriation buffer: McCoys 5A medium supplemented with 5% (v/v) fetal calf serum (FCS) and 5 nM 2-naphthol-6,8-disulfonic acid (NDA)

0.025% (w/v) trypsin in elutriation buffer

0.002% (w/v) DNase I in elutriation buffer

10% (v/v) FCS

0.9% saline

70% ethanol or 6% hydrogen peroxide

Confluent cell monolayer

Protocol

1. Aspirate culture medium (supernatant) from flasks.

2. Wash cells with 0.9% saline. Aspirate saline.

3. Remove the cells carefully from the culture flask with 0.025% (w/v) trypsin and 0.002% (w/v) DNase I.

4. Once release of cells is complete, add medium containing 10% (v/v) FCS.

5. Examine the cell suspension under a phase-contrast microscope for cell clumping. If this is evident, then disrupt them by vigorous pipeting through a Pasteur pipet.

6. Pellet the cells at 150 g for 5 min. Resuspend in less than 20 ml of medium containing 10% (v/v) FCS.

7. Set-up the elutriation system as described in *Protocol 3.1*. Set the rotor speed to 1525 r.p.m., and the load cells at flow rate 9.4 ml min^{-1}.

8. Once the cells are loaded, run 75–100 ml of the eluate to waste while the cells equilibrate within the chamber.

9. Collect 12 separate fractions of 50–75 ml by increasing the flow rate using 1.4-ml increments.

10. Stop the centrifuge and collect any cells and aggregates remaining in the chamber as they wash out.

11. Centrifuge each fraction. Resuspend in desired volume and remove aliquots for viability, counting or analysis.

Notes

Method based on that described by Meistrich et al. (1977).

If required, the elutriation chamber, tubing, and rotor head can be sterilized using 70% ethanol or 6% (v/v) H_2O_2 as described in *Protocol 3.1*.

Protocol 3.3

Purification of rat hepatocyte couplets

Equipment

Sterile scalpel and forceps

Petri dishes

150-µm pore nylon gauze

Centrifuge rotor

Phase-contrast microscope

Collection/centrifuge tubes

Reagents

Hanks balance salt solution (HBSS)

Ca-free HBSS

0.03% (w/v) Collagenase (Type A) in HBSS

Krebs–Henseleit solution

Elutriation buffer: Krebs–Henseleit solution gassed and stored at 19°C, supplemented with 0.1% (w/v) glucose and 0.1% (w/v) BSA

Leibowitz-15 tissue culture medium

0.4% (w/v) Trypan blue solution in saline

Protocol

1. Pre-perfuse rat liver *in situ* for 10 min using Ca-free HBSS followed by a 4-min perfusion in HBSS containing 0.03% (w/v) collagenase.

2. Excise liver and plunge into ice-cold Krebs–Henseleit buffer. Finely chop and stir to release the cells.

3. Filter the resulting suspension of cells and debris through 150-µm pore nylon gauze. Allow to settle by gravity sedimentation.

4. Wash the cells twice by settling before the elutriation process.

5. Set up the elutriatior as described in *Protocol 3.1* using a small standard chamber mounted in a JE-5.0 rotor head and a J6-MB centrifuge. Using a rotor speed of 1100 r.p.m., load the sample at an elutriation buffer flow rate of 10 ml min^{-1}.

6. Ensure that all the cells are loaded by gently agitating the loading chamber.

7. Once all the cells are loaded, bypass the loading chamber and allow the eluate to run to waste for at least 10 min.

8. Increase the flow rate to 20 ml min⁻¹ and again discard the eluate which will contain the majority of nonviable cells and cell debris from the loaded suspension.

9. Increase the buffer flow rate in increments of 5 ml min⁻¹. Collect 100-ml fractions at each increment and keep on ice.

10. Centrifuge the fractions at 85 *g* for 5 min. Resuspend in culture medium.

11. Determine the cell population and assess viability by Trypan blue exclusion.

Notes

Method based on that described by Wilton *et al.* (1991).

Hanks balance salt solution (HBSS): 137 mM NaCl, 26 mM NaHCO$_3$, 0.6 mM Na$_2$HPO$_4$, 5.4 mM KCl, 0.4 mM KH$_2$PO$_4$, 4 mM CaCl$_2$, and 5.6 mM glucose – gas the solution at 19°C with 95%/5% O$_2$/CO$_2$ for 20 min, and correct the pH to 7.45.

Krebs–Henseleit solution: 118 mM NaCl , 4.8 mM KCl, 1.2 mM MgSO$_4$, 1 mM KH$_2$PO$_4$, 24 mM NaHCO$_3$, and 3.2 mM CaCl$_2$ – gas the solution at 4°C with 95%/5% O$_2$/CO$_2$, correct the pH to 7.45 and store at 4°C.

The temperature should be maintained at 19°C throughout the run.

Count the cells using phase-contrast microscopy and adjust to an appropriate concentration prior to loading using elutriation buffer. Optimally a volume of approximately 15–20 ml is used to load 2×10^8 cells.

Where the rotor is maintained at a constant speed and the rate of flow of the buffer through the chamber is increased, the small (single) cells elute first, followed sequentially by the couplets, the triplets and finally the larger multiples.

Chapter 4

Free-flow electrophoresis

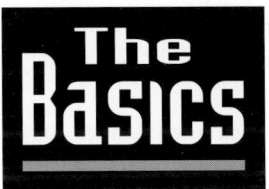

1. Introduction

Techniques, such as electrophoretic separation, of cell separation based upon properties of the cell surface often permit a high degree of purification of the separated cell population. The majority of cells carry a net surface negative charge at physiological pH. The intensity of this surface charge density varies for different cell types and thus allows separation of the different types by rate of migration in an electric field. Separation is based upon differences in electrophoretic mobility.

The density of surface charge does not directly reflect the electrochemical composition at the cell surface since, in an ionic medium, a layer of counter ions (ions of opposite charge) surrounds the cell forming an electric double layer. Some of these positive ions neutralize cell membrane charge moieties. The electrokinetic or 'zeta' potential is the potential at the outer region of this double layer and therefore represents the apparent cell surface charge. Electrophoretic mobility depends upon this 'zeta' potential.

Four basic electrophoretic methods have been used for cell separation; free-flow electrophoresis (FFE), density gradient electrophoresis, endless belt electrophoresis and stable-flow-free boundary electrophoresis (STAFLO). Of these, FFE is widely used today. In FFE, an accurately controlled flow of buffer and cells pass downwards through an electric field. As the cells flow down in the stream of buffer they are deflected toward the anode and the amount of deflection (electrophoretic mobility) is proportional to their 'zeta' potential. The deflected cells collect into a series of tubes.

As the electrophoresis separation normally occurs in a continuous flowing buffer that exceeds 1 g sedimentation, the size or density of the cell is not normally influential in the separation. Hence, FFE is particularly useful in separating cells that differ only very slightly in size or density from one another. Once separated and collected the cells can undergo further analysis. While FFE is commonly employed to further separate purified cells into subpopulations that differ in net surface charge characteristics, it can also be exploited to monitor changes in the electrophoretic mobility of a single population of cells that have been treated in some way (e.g. metabolically activated, neuraminidase treated or surface labeled).

The extent to which a cell is deflected towards the anode as a function of its surface 'zeta' potential, the applied electrical field and the rate of buffer flow is described by the following equation:

$$\text{Apparent electrophoretic mobility } U = \frac{l \times A \times K}{I \times t} \qquad (4.1)$$

where: l=migration distance (cm), A=cross-sectional area of chamber (cm^2), K=specific conductivity of medium (Siemens cm^{-1}), I=current (A), t=residence time in chamber (s):

$$t = \frac{2 \times Vk}{3 \times Qk} \qquad (4.2)$$

where: Vk = chamber volume (cm^3) and Qk = chamber flow rate (cm^3 s^{-1}).

FFE can achieve a high cell recovery and viability. As long as the cells do not aggregate for any reason during their passage through the separation chamber, 90% cell recovery should be attainable.

2.   Main types of FFE equipment

2.1   Elphor VAP

FFE was originally developed by Kurt Hannig in the early 1960s, resulting in the commercial production of the Elphor Vap apparatus by Bender Hobein, which is the most extensively used cell electrophoresis apparatus.

The separation chamber consists of a mirrored glass inner and plastic outer chamber wall, forming a chamber 50 cm high, 10 cm wide, with a 0.05 cm gap between them, down which a continuous flow of chamber buffer passes from a reservoir placed on top of the chamber. The chamber buffer flows down between the two electrode compartments and exits through 96 ports into collection tubes. The flow rate of the chamber buffer is controlled by a peristaltic pump.

The sample is introduced into the system via the sample injection unit situated on top of the chamber unit. It incorporates a glass Hamilton syringe within a cooling chamber that also rotates to maintain the cells in suspension during their passage into the chamber. A second syringe is connected to the sample syringe. The second syringe drawn by a syringe pump controls the sample injection rate into the downward flowing chamber buffer. The sample can enter the chamber from one of four desired inlet ports of entry across the chamber.

The control unit regulates chamber and electrode buffer flow rates, temperature, and the voltage and current applied across the separation chamber. It also houses reservoirs of electrode buffer media which are transported to the electrode compartments which border both edges of the separation chamber. The continual circulation of the electrode buffer over the electrodes minimizes changes in pH and ionic composition of the buffer. Various safety circuits informing the operator of electrical and fluid leaks, overheating, or surges in current or voltage, also comprise the control unit.

The cooling system pumps cooler fluid behind the mirrored plate in the sample chamber. The heat generated by the electrical current during electrophoretic separation is removed rapidly and efficiently by the cooling fluid, preventing disturbance of the laminar flow. The temperature can be set between 4° and 37°C.

2.2 OCTOPUS-PZE

An alternative to the VAP instruments is the OCTOPUS-PZE FFE apparatus. This instrument borrows several design features from the VAP machines. While not dissimilar in appearance to the VAP 22, the OCTOPUS-PZE is more compact. The dimensions of the separation chamber are the same as that used in the VAP 22, as is the capacity for 96 fractions to be collected. However the separation procedure does differ in some unique ways. For instance, the cell sample and chamber buffer are delivered into the separation chamber from the bottom of the chamber rather than the top. The separation medium flow upwards is controlled by a manifold pump. Secondly, a counterflow medium is introduced at the top of the chamber, the counterflow action ensures good mixing of the separation medium, enhancing separation. Thirdly, cell separation on the basis of differences in surface zeta potential is enhanced still further by the infusion of a high conductivity–stabilization medium, which is allowed to run parallel to the electrodes within the separation chamber.

3. Buffers

A number of buffers have been developed with the aim of maintaining cell viability while enhancing the separation resolution. Some of the most common buffers used to separate cells by FFE are described. As no one buffer is best for all applications, it is wise to check and optimize the buffer system of choice to suit the cells to be separated.

3.1 Separation chamber buffers

It is important that the cells are suspended in a medium that allows the cells to remain in a stable state and at a concentration that will prevent cell clumping. As with most cell separation techniques, the cells to be separated must be in a good physical and metabolic state. If the cells of interest have not been separated by FFE before, they should be suspended in the chosen separation buffer for periods of time and an aspect(s) of their functional or biochemical status monitored. Such steps are taken to ensure that the buffer does not in any way affect any of the cell's metabolic pathways that may be assayed after separation.

Low ionic media

Low ionic strength buffers are routinely used for cell separation by electrophoresis in order to obtain a high voltage with a low heat production. Irrespective of the cell type to be separated, most low ionic buffers are triethanolamine-based. The buffer should be of physiological pH between 7.0 and 7.4, and osmolality within the range 0.28–0.33 Osmol; osmolality is normally maintained within this range by adding glycine, glucose, sucrose or an alternative nonionic sugar. The conductivity should be between 200 and 800 μS cm^{-1}; the lower end of this range is more common. Examples of commonly used sample chamber and electrode buffers are listed in *Table 4.1*. Generally, sugar-based buffers containing low concentrations of triethanolamine and a pH of 7.2–7.4 are suitable for most separations; they have not been reported to impair cell function. Nevertheless, exposure of

Table 4.1. Examples of separation chamber and electrode buffers used in VAP instruments

Cell type	Separation chamber buffer	Electrode buffer	Ref.
Platelets	10 mM Triethanolamine 280 mM Glycine	100 mM Triethanolamine	Crook et al. (1992)
Lymphocytes	15 mM Triethanolamine 4 mM Potassium acetate 240 mM Glycine 11 mM Glucose	75 mM Triethanolamine 20 mM Potassium acetate	Heidrich and Hannig (1989)
Neutrophils	280 mM Triethanolamine 30 mM Glucose	100 mM Triethanolamine	Eggleton et al. (1992)
Kidney proximal tubule	210 mM Sucrose 100 mM Glycine 4 mM Na_2HPO_4 1 mM NaH_2PO_4 5 mM Glucose 1 mM $CaCl_2$ 0.025 mM $MgCl_2$ 5 mg l^{-1} BSA	100 mM Triethanolamine	Toutain et al. (1989)
Malarial parasites	10 mM Triethanolamine 10 mM Acetic acid 0.1 mM $MgSO_4$ 250 mM Sucrose	110 mM Triethanolamine 110 mM Acetic acid	Heidrich et al. (1979)

cells to triethanolamine-based buffers should be kept to a minimum. Standard FFE buffers have been shown to buffer poorly at the pH employed in most separations and it has been recommended that zwitterionic buffers are used instead. Once cells have been separated, they should be quickly fractionated, washed and removed from the chamber buffer of choice.

Triethanolamine-free media

There is some debate over the use of chloride ions in buffers; for instance, when sodium chloride is used, the chloride ions are changed by electrical current into hypochlorite, which is toxic to cells. On the other hand the inclusion of 50 mM calcium has been suggested to enhance cell separation. Yet such media have been used in the OCTOPUS-PZE process. The media, which comprises of a sodium chloride-based buffered saline, combines the use of iso-osmolal glucose, glycine and sucrose in the volume ratio 1:1.3:1:0.7 respectively and avoids altogether the use of triethanolamine.

3.2   Electrode chamber buffers

The electrode buffers are contained within the channels of the electrode chambers behind filter membranes, and do not come into contact with cells. Therefore, the conductivity of the buffer is more critical than the osmolality. Normally, electrode buffers with conductivity five to ten times greater than the separation buffers are used in order to supply sufficient ions to aid separation of the cells as they pass down through the separation chamber.

Table 4.2. Composition of electrode and stabilization buffers used in the OCTOPUS-PZE instrument

	Electrode buffer		Stabilization buffer	
	g l⁻¹	mM	g l⁻¹	mM
Anodal media				
Phosphoric acid	19.6	200	9.8	100
Glycine			5.6	75
Sucrose			17.1	50
Cathodal media				
Tris–HCl	23.6	150	11.8	75
NaCl	8.8	150	4.4	75
Glycine			5.6	75
Sucrose			17.1	50

Anodal and cathodal media are adjusted to pH 7.4 with NaOH and HCl, respectively.

As exemplified by *Table 4.1*, most workers have employed electrode buffers that are triethanolamine based for use in VAP instruments.

As noted earlier, the OCTOPUS-PZE process employs a third buffer called the 'stabilization' buffer. The use of stabilization media allows a more homogeneous supply of ions in the area near the membranes inside the separation chamber, which in turn improves separation of cells. It reduces/prevents fluctuations in ion concentrations at the intersection between the electrode and cell separation chamber.

The electrode and stabilization media are custom designed for use with each individual electrode, and unlike the electrode buffers used in the VAP instruments, they do not contain ethanolamine (*Table 4.2*).

4. Preparation of cell samples for FFE

4.1 Types of cells separated by FFE

A number of diverse cell types have been successfully separated by FFE (*Table 4.3*). FFE has been used mostly to study blood cells, which reflects the initial ease by which these cells can be isolated by standard density gradient techniques (Chapter 2). However, cells from other tissues are often obtained by mechanical disruption, enzymatic treatment or a combination of both (Chapter 1). This can lead to changes in the cell surface, be it charge or receptor status, and overall protein composition. These changes may interfere with the subsequent electrokinetic properties of the cell surface membrane upon separation by FFE. Nevertheless, a number of laboratories have successfully employed FFE to study fibroblasts (Lieser *et al.*, 1989), hepatocytes (Evers *et al.*, 1989), and kidney cells (Toutain *et al.*, 1989). In addition, protozoa, bacteria, and tumor or immortal cell lines have been studied.

4.2 Purification and preparation of cell samples before FFE

Depending on the objectives of a particular experiment, the choice of a particular cell preparation technique is important. For example, in cell heterogeneity studies, the initial purification step must provide high yields of cells.

Table 4.3. Application of free-flow electrophoresis (FFE) to study various cell types

Cell type	Ref.	Cell type	Ref.
Blood		*Germline*	
Platelets	Crook *et al.* (1992); Wilson and Graham (1986)	Spermatozoa	Engelmann *et al.* (1988)
Lymphocytes	Hansen and Hannig (1982); Hansen *et al.* (1989)	*Tumor cells*	
		Ehrlich ascites	Mayhew (1968)
Monocytes	Bauer and Hannig (1984)	Mast cell ascites	Pretlow *et al.* (1981)
Neutrophils	Eggleton *et al.* (1992)	Leukemic	Schubert *et al.* (1973)
Erythrocytes	Hannig *et al.* (1990)	*Protozoa*	
Bone marrow	Zeiller and Hansen (1979)	*Plasmodium* sp.	Heidrich *et al.* (1979)
Somatic		Trypanosomes	Siddiqui *et al.* (1990)
Fibroblasts	Lieser *et al.* (1989)		
Hepatocytes	Ali *et al.* (1989)	*Prokaryotic*	
Kidney	Toutain *et al.* (1989)	*Escherichia coli*	Holzenburg *et al.* (1989)
		Staphylococcus aureus	Ramsey *et al.* (1980)
		Streptococci sp.	Uhlenbruck *et al.* (1988)

In studies in which cells differ very little in any physical characteristics, subsequent modification of the surface of the cells is required before FFE is undertaken. This can be achieved by labeling the cells of interest with monoclonal antibodies specific for one subset of cells. Antibodies have a lower net negative charge than cell membranes, and consequently, labeling cells with immunoglobulins lowers the electrophoretic mobility of the cells, allowing resolution of the two or more populations of cells.

Once purified, cell preparations can be suspended in media commonly used to maintain the cells such as phosphate-buffered saline (PBS) or Hank's balanced salt solution (HBSS) without calcium and magnesium. Alternatively, they can be placed in sample buffer and adjusted to the appropriate concentration just prior to electrophoresis.

Protocols 4.1–4.5 describe methods used to prepare cells for fractionation by FFE.

5.   FFE of cell samples

5.1   Preparation of FFE apparatus

The FFE instrument manual should be consulted for preparing the apparatus. A step-by-step guide is provided by the manufacturers and should be followed carefully. In brief, prepare fresh chamber and electrode buffers, and fill appropriate reservoirs. A short cell-free pre-run should be performed to check for leaks and power surges. The machine can then be prepared for cell separation. The manuals will also give information on the precise choice of flow rates to ensure both good and reproducible separation of cells. A guide to settings for chamber buffer flow rates and voltage commonly used for a number of different cell types using the VAP apparatus is given in *Table 4.4*.

Table 4.4. Examples of chamber buffer flow rates and voltage commonly used during separation by FFE using VAP apparatus

Cell type	Flow rates (ml h^{-1})	V cm^{-1}	Ref.
Lymphocytes	550	118	Heidrich and Hannig (1989)
Platelets	500	130	Crook et al. (1992)
Neutrophils	405	90–100	Eggleton et al. (1992)
Kidney	180	170	Toutain et al. (1989)
Malarial parasites	180	135	Heidrich et al. (1979)

5.2   Construction of cell fractionation profiles

As the cells separate in the chamber on the basis of differences in electrokinetic properties, they form a broad band covering an area of 1–20 fractions. On leaving the chamber they pass through 10–20 of the 96 silica tubes located at the base of the chamber, and are collected either in plastic collection tubes or in two 48-well microtiter plates. The location of the cells is determined using hemocytometer counts or turbidity measurements in a spectrophotometer at either 500 or 280 nm.

Biochemical and functional analysis of the separated cells as subpopulations can be achieved by either assaying every individual fraction, or pooling the cells as three or four subpopulations of equal number. One method commonly used to prepare the cells as subpopulations is that described as follows. As shown in *Figure 4.1* a cell profile can be subdivided as three subpopulations, the least electronegative (A), the median (B) and the most electronegative (C). The least and most electronegative subpopulations are selected by bisecting the profile at the point that represents 50% of the total cell population recovered. Lines are drawn perpendicular to these intersecting points, and the cells pooled from the selected areas under the curve. Generally the least and most electronegative cells populations each

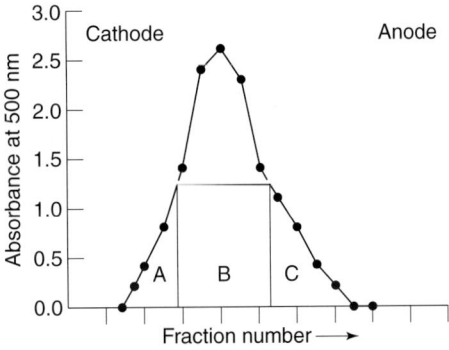

Figure 4.1

Subdivision of cells into subpopulations after free-flow electrophoresis. The cell profile is divided into three populations, (A) the least electronegative, (B) the median population and (C) the most electropositive population.

represent about 15–20% of the total cells recovered, while the median fraction contains approximately 60–70% of the cells.

5.3   Evaluation of cells separated by FFE

Once cells have been separated by FFE it is wise to check that the cells have indeed been separated on the basis of real and reproducible electrokinetic differences. This is achieved by re-electrophoresis of pools of isolated cell subpopulations. Subpopulations of cells collected from each end of the first profile upon re-electrophoresis are mixed and separated once more. Each pool of cells should relocate at a peak position coinciding with the same population of cells in the original separation (*Protocol 4.6*). Yet, it is best to perform such separations on fixed cells so as to avoid any changes in membrane characteristics during the procedure, which may occur by passing live cells through the chamber more than once.

6.   Factors affecting FFE

6.1   Cell clumping

Although FFE is an excellent separation technique for blood cells, most types of blood cells are prone to aggregation during separation. Changes in temperature, pH, isotonicity, and *g* forces may lead to cell clumping or aggregate formation. While most of these factors are not a problem during FFE, as the technique is a gentle one, and the parameters can be adjusted to maintain the cells in a labile state, the maintenance of a highly concentrated suspension of cells in the sample syringe, or their passage through a narrow bore syringe into the separation chamber can sometimes result in cell clumping. Cell clumping will adversely affect the separation resolution and so where such problems exist, it is recommended that the cells be suspended in chamber buffer containing a protease cocktail. For instance, in the case of neutrophils, a cocktail of DNase, leupeptin and PMSF should be used. Also, cells prepared from tissues by enzymatic digestion should be filtered to remove debris and aggregates.

6.2   Leaks

Leaks occur most commonly at sites where the buffer and sample tubes leave and enter the separation chamber, and between the tubing connections between the electrode buffer reservoir and the electrode compartment. The separation chamber is sealed with double gaskets to prevent leakage from the chamber itself, this is an important safety feature, as leakage of fluid from this area while the chamber is in use may result in high voltage electrical arching between the electrodes. If a leak occurs in the separation chamber while an actual separation is in progress, the separation will have to be stopped and the chamber temperature brought up to approximately 15°C before all power can be turned off and the leak repaired. Another potential site of leakage is between the electrode compartment and the medium in the separation chamber. Leakage of one fluid into the region of the other will lead to voltage fluctuation and the efficacy of cell separation will be adversely affected.

Needless to say, regular maintenance of the apparatus and all tubing will prevent any such leaks occurring during separation. Furthermore, before beginning any separation, check that all major tubing is connected correctly. It is good practice to pre-run the machine for at least 15 min before addition of the sample to check for any leaks.

6.3   Bacterial contamination and blockages

The FFE apparatus and tubing are prone to bacterial contamination and blockage caused by cell aggregation or salt deposits and so must be cleaned and kept unblocked during a FFE run. A number of precautions can be performed to eliminate or avoid such contamination. They include regular cleaning with Teepol or similar mild detergent. Other precautions include the removal of all cell separation media immediately after use, and regular flushing of the apparatus with sterile distilled water. It is difficult to keep all parts of the FFE apparatus completely sterile. However, if sterile conditions are required, then the separation chamber, buffer supply reservoirs, and all tubing can be treated with 3.7% formaldehyde solution for 1–2 h. All formaldehyde-treated apparatus should then be thoroughly rinsed with sterile endotoxin-free distilled water. Formaldehyde, however, will shorten the life of the tubing.

6.4   Temperature

For many cell separations it is desirable to maintain the cells and the separation chamber between 4° and 6°C. If for any reason a circuit overload occurs, the current is shut off automatically as a safety control. This can lead to a rapid cooling of the separation chamber to an unfavorable temperature. If the drop in temperature is severe, the back plate of the chamber may crack and break. Therefore it is imperative to immediately switch off the cooling circuit to prevent further refrigeration and to discover the underlying fault. The most common cause of circuit overload and shut-off is leakage of separation or electrode buffer from their respective chambers. In addition, faulty membranes, thermosensors or incorrect maintenance of the apparatus can result in such problems. If possible, get the power to come back on and increase the current to help warm the plate. In addition, the flow rate can also be reduced to impair heat loss and help warm the plate.

6.5   pH and conductivity

If fluctuations in current or voltage are observed during a cell separation run and/or the cell profiles are not as well resolved as usual, there may be a problem with the separation or electrode buffer. Simple but routine steps should be performed to avoid such problems. It is wise to always prepare both electrode and separation buffer on the day of use, or at most, the evening before, and store at 4°C. It is also important to check the pH, osmolality and conductivity of each buffer before use. Indeed, some buffers have been shown to change in property during separation (Rodkey, 1990) and so it is necessary to check the buffer of choice before electrophoresis of cells. Checks should be made of the buffer in a cell-free electrophoresis run; samples taken at the anodal and cathodal ends of the separation chamber as well as intermediate fractions should be compared with the original buffer.

6.6 Filter membranes

If the FFE apparatus is not being used routinely, it is often best to wash and drain the separation and electrode chamber of all fluid, to prevent bacterial contamination. However, this will lead to drying out of the filter membranes and consequently the deterioration of the membranes. Therefore the membranes should be removed and stored in a mild antibacterial solution, such as 2–5% formaldehyde solution until required. When required, the membranes should be thoroughly rinsed in distilled water or a small quantity of 70% ethyl alcohol followed by water. Cellulose acetate membranes are available which are more resistant to drying out and microorganism contamination.

7. Applications of FFE

FFE is used to separate cells into subpopulations by exploiting differences in cell surface charge. It is not recommended that FFE is used to separate individual cells that possess gross morphological or functional differences, when simpler and less expensive density gradient techniques (Chapter 2) will suffice. Though, isolation of cells by gradient density techniques prior to FFE is recommended to remove gross contamination of other cell types. FFE can then be used to separate cells on the basis of differences in electrokinetic properties alone, as is the case in isolation of subpopulations of human neutrophils and spermatozoa, or in combination with immunological techniques to isolate pure populations of B and T lymphocytes. The FFE apparatus is capable of separating cells that differ by as little as 5–10% in electrophoretic mobility. A selection of cells separated by FFE is given in *Table 4.3*.

However, FFE should not be thought of as purely a separation technique, it can be used to study changes in electrokinetic properties of the membranes of whole cells. For instance, the major contributor of surface electronegative charge on many cells is believed to be sialic acid moieties associated with the membrane glycoproteins. By incubating the cells with the enzyme neuraminidase (0.1–0.5 U ml^{-1} per 10^7 cells), for 60 min at 37°C, terminal labile sialic acid residues are cleaved from the outer surface from the cell membrane. Cells with and without neuraminidase treatment can then be fractionated by FFE. Changes in cell surface charge often reflect modification or alteration of membrane-associated processes.

FFE has also been used to separate a number of cell types into subpopulations to investigate the relationship between their surface membrane electrokinetic properties and various resting and stimulated states, that is, to study biochemical differences in cell subpopulations. One such example is the fractionation of neutrophils. Neutrophils possess many stimulant motile activities, such as adhesion, chemotactic migration, phagocytosis, secretion of granule-stored constituents and so on, which require reorganization of certain elements of the plasma membrane–cytoskeleton axis. Separation into subpopulations by FFE has revealed that the least and most electronegative cells differ in electrophoretic mobilities that range between 1.04 and 1.18 μm s^{-1}V^{-1}cm^{-1}, respectively. Yet more interestingly, biochemical differences are also evident, the least electronegative cells generally phagocytose bacteria and generate superoxide after stimulation at twice the rate of the most electronegative cells separated by FFE (Eggleton *et al.,* 1992).

References

Ali, N., Milligan, G. and Evans, W.H. (1989) G-proteins of rat liver membranes. *Mol. Cell. Biochem.* **91**: 75–84.

Bauer, J. and Hannig, K. (1984) Electrophoretic characterization of human monocytes and lymphocytes before and after stimulation with concavalin A. *Electrophoresis* **5**: 155–159.

Crook, M. and Crawford, N. (1989) Electrokinetic, analytical, and functional heterogeneity of circulating human platelets. *Biochim. Biophys. Acta* **1014**: 26–39.

Crook, M., Machin, S. and Crawford, N. (1992) Electrokinetic behaviour and surface sialic acid status of blood platelets in essential thrombocythaemia (ET). *Eur. J. Haematol.* **49**: 128–132.

Eggleton, P., Gargan, R. and Fisher, D. (1989) Rapid method for the isolation of neutrophils in high yield without the use of dextran or gradient polymers. *J. Immunol. Methods* **121**: 105–113.

Eggleton, P., Fisher, D. and Crawford, N. (1992) Heterogeneity in the circulating neutrophil pool. *J. Leuk. Biol.* **51**: 617–625.

Engelmann, U., Krassmigg, F., Schatz, H. and Schill, W.B. (1988) Separation of human X and Y spermatozoa by free-flow electrophoresis. *Gamete Res.* **19**: 151–160.

Evers, C., Meiter, P.J. and Murer, H. (1989) Separation of hepatocyte plasma membrane domains by free-flow electrophoresis. *Anal. Biochem.* **176**: 338–343.

Hannig, K., Kowalski, M., Klock, G., Zimmerman, U. and Mang, V. (1990) Free-flow electrophoresis under microgravity. *Electrophoresis* **11**: 600–604.

Hansen, E. and Hannig, K. (1982) Antigen-specific electrophoretic cell separation. *J. Immunol. Methods* **51**: 197–208.

Hansen, E., Wustrow, T.P. and Hannig, K. (1989) Antigen-specific electrophoretic cell separation for immunological investigations. *Electrophoresis* **10**: 645–652.

Heidrich, H.G. and Hannig, K. (1989) In *Methods in Enzymology* (eds S. Fleischer and B. Fleischer). Academic Press, London, New York, Vol. 171, pp. 513–533.

Heidrich, H.G., Russmann, L., Bayer, B. and Jung, A. (1979) Free-flow electrophoresis for the separation of malaria infected and uninfected mouse erythrocytes and for the isolation of free parasites (*Plasmodium vinckei*). *Z. Parasitenkd.* **58**: 151–159.

Holzenburg, A., Engel, A., Kessler, R., Manz, H.J., Lustig, A. and Aebi, U. (1989) Rapid isolation of OmpF porin-LPS complexes suitable for structure–function studies. *Biochemistry* **28**: 4187–4193.

Kreisberg, J.I., Sachs, G., Pretlow, T.G. and McCuire, R.A. (1977) *J. Cell Physiol.* **93**: 169.

Lieser, M., Harma, E., Kern, H., Bach, G. and Cantz, M. (1989) Ganglioside GM3 sialidase activity in fibroblasts of normal individuals and of patients with sialidosis and mucolipidosis IV. *Biochem. J.* **260**: 69.

Mayhew, E. (1968) Electrophoretic mobility of Ehrlich ascites carcinoma cells grown *in vitro* and *in vivo*. *Cancer Res.* **28**: 1590–1595.

Pretlow, T.P., Stewart, H.B., Sachs, G., Pretlow, T.G. and Pitts, A.M. (1981) Free-flow electrophoresis of an ascites mast-cell tumour. *Br. J. Cancer* **43**: 537–541.

Ramsey, W.S., Nowlan, E.D. and Simpson, L.B. (1980) *Eur. J. Appl. Microbiol.* **9**: 217.

Rodkey, L.S. (1990) Free-flow cell electrophoresis using zwitterionic buffer. *Appl. Theor. Electrophoresis* **1**: 243–247.

Schubert, J.C.F., Walther, F., Holzberg, E., Pasher, G. and Zeiller, K. (1973) Preparative electrophoretic separation of normal and neoplastic human bone marrow cells. *Klin. Wschr.* **51**: 327–332.

Siddiqui, A.A., Zhou, Y., Podesta, R.B. and Clarke, M.W. (1990) Isolation of a highly enriched plasma membrane fraction of *Trypanosoma brucei* by free-flow electrophoresis. *Mol. Biochem. Parasitol.* **40**: 95–103.

Toutain, H., Fillastre, J.P. and Morin, J.P. (1989) Preparative free-flow electrophoresis for the isolation of two populations of proximal cells from the rabbit kidney. *Eur. J. Cell Biol.* **49**: 274–280.

Uhlenbruck, G., Froml, A., Lutticken, R. and Hannig, K. (1988) Cell electrophoresis of group B streptococci. *Zbl. Bakt. Hyg.* **A 270**: 28–34.

Wilson, R.B.J. and Graham, J.M. (1986) Isolation of platelets from human blood by free-flow electrophoresis. *Clin. Chim. Acta* **159**: 211–217.

Zeiller, K. and Hansen, E. (1979) Characterization of rat bone marrow cells. *Cell. Immunol.* **44**: 381–394.

Protocol 4.1

Purification and preparation of lymphocytes for FFE (Hansen *et al.*, 1989)

Equipment

Bench-top centrifuge

Glass beads

Gauze

Centrifuge tubes

Pipets

Reagents

Ficoll-Hypaque

Puck G

Density gradient medium (density 1.077 g ml^{-1}, e.g. MSL from Nycomed Amersham)

Monoclonal antibody OKT8 and OKT4

Rabbit ant-human IgM antiserum

Tetrarhodamine isothiocyanate (TRITC)-conjugated goat anti-rabbit IgG immunoglobulin and rabbit anti-mouse IgG immunoglobulin

Sample chamber buffer

Protocol

1. Collect 200 ml human peripheral blood and defibrinate by gentle shaking in 50 ml tubes with 20 glass beads.

2. Remove the clot by filtration through gauze.

3. Centrifuge the cells at 200 *g* for 10 min at room temperature, and discard the platelet containing supernatant.

4. To prepare lymphocyte-rich cells by Ficoll-Hypaque density centrifugation, resuspend the cells in three volumes of Puck G. Layer two volumes of cells on top of one volume density gradient medium (density 1.077 g ml^{-1}) and centrifuge at 400 *g* for 30 min at room temperature. Harvest the cell band and wash three times in cold Puck G medium by centrifugation for 10 min at 100 *g*. Concentrate the lymphocytes to 5 × 10^7 cells ml^{-1}.

5. Maintain cells at 4°C and incubate for 20 min with the appropriate dilutions of either rabbit anti-human IgM to identify B lymphocytes; mouse anti-human OKT8 to label CD8+ T cells; mouse anti-human OKT4 to label CD4+ cells.

6. Wash cells twice in Puck G at 100 **g** for 7 min.

7. Label the appropriate cells using secondary antibody (tetrarhodamine isothiocyanate (TRITC)-conjugated goat anti-rabbit and rabbit anti-mouse IgG immunoglobulin) for 20 min at 4°C.

8. Wash cells twice in Puck G at 100 **g** for 7 min.

9. Adjust the cell concentration to 5×10^7 cells ml^{-1}, maintain the antibody treated cells at 4°C, and place in sample chamber buffer before FFE.

Protocol 4.2

Purification and preparation of platelets for FFE (Crook and Crawford, 1989)

Equipment

Bench-top centrifuge

Centrifuge tubes

Pipets

Reagents

CDP-adenine

Citrate buffer: 36 mM citric acid, 5 mM glucose, 5 mM KCl, 90 mM NaCl, 10 mM EDTA, adjusted to pH 6.5 with NaOH

Taxol

Sample chamber buffer

Protocol

1. Centrifuge 60 ml of CDP-adenine anticoagulated whole blood at 120 g for 20 min at room temperature.

2. Harvest the platelet-rich plasma.

3. Resuspend the remaining red cell layer in citrate buffer to the original whole blood volume and centrifuge as before. Harvest the supernatant containing additional platelets and add to the platelet-rich plasma pool. Repeat this procedure once more.

4. Resuspend platelets in citrate buffer to a cell volume ratio of 1:3 and wash twice.

5. Resuspend cells in citrate buffer containing 10^{-5} M taxol to help maintain their discoidicity, for 25–30 min.

6. Wash the cells in citrate buffer to remove excess taxol, and then resuspend the platelets in chamber buffer before FFE.

Note

Ensure yield of platelets is in the order of 90–95%, which is greater than that achieved by conventionally prepared platelet-rich plasma techniques (approximately 70%).

Protocol 4.3

Purification and preparation of neutrophils for FFE (Eggleton *et al.*, 1989)

Equipment

Bench-top centrifuge

Centrifuge tubes

Pipets

Reagents

Isotonic ammonium chloride

HBSS

EDTA

Sample chamber buffer

Protocol

1. Mix one volume of EDTA (1.5 mg ml^{-1} blood) anticoagulated whole blood with four volumes cold (4°C) isotonic ammonium chloride, mix, and leave for 15 min to permit erythrocyte hemolysis.

2. Pellet the leucocytes at 160 **g** for 10 min. Discard the supernatant.

3. Resuspend the leucocytes in 10 ml HBSS and centrifuge at 5 **g** for 10 min. Discard the supernatant and repeat wash.

4. Resuspend the cells in chamber buffer prior to use.

Note

This method produces a substantially higher yield of neutrophils than either dextran sedimentation (50% yield) or dextran sedimentation and Ficoll-Hypaque centrifugation combined (15–20% yield) generate. The yield of resulting neutrophils should be in the order of 70% and approximately 80% pure.

Protocol 4.4

Purification and preparation of kidney cells for FFE (Kreisberg *et al.*, 1977)

Equipment

Sterile scalpel and forceps

Petri dish

Bench-top centrifuge

Nitex (36 µm)

Centrifuge tubes

Pipets

Reagents

10% fetal calf serum (FCS) in MEM

0.25% trypsin in MEM

HBSS

HBSS with 5 U ml^{-1} heparin

Sample chamber buffer

Protocol

1. Perfuse rat kidneys with HBSS containing 5 U ml^{-1} heparin, excise and remove the papillae.

2. Take the remaining tissue and mince to fragments of 1–2 mm.

3. Agitate fragments for 10 min each in three changes of MEM containing 10% FCS. Discard the supernatants from the wash fluids after allowing the tissue to settle.

4. Disaggregate the kidney fragments in ten times 50-ml changes of MEM containing 0.25% trypsin at room temperature of 20-min durations.

5. Collect the cells from the third to tenth trypsin supernatants, cool to 4°C and recover the cells at 97 *g* for 8 min.

6. Filter cells through a layer of Nitex (36 µm) to remove aggregates.

7. Adjust cell concentration to 1–2 × 10^7 cells ml^{-1} in sample chamber buffer and maintain cells at 4°C until separated.

Protocol 4.5

Purification and preparation of ascitic human cells for FFE (Pretlow *et al.*, 1981)

Equipment

Bench-top centrifuge

Nitex (48 μm)

Centrifuge tubes

Pipets

Reagents

10% FCS in MEM

Sample chamber buffer

Protocol

1. Harvest ascitic tumors from the peritoneal cavity of mice by repeated washing with 3-ml aliquots of 10% FCS in MEM at 4°C.

2. Centrifuge the cells at 97 **g** for 8 min at 4°C.

3. Wash three times in FFE sample chamber buffer and adjust cell concentration to $1–2 \times 10^7$ cells ml^{-1}.

4. Filter cells through a layer of Nitex (48 μm) to remove aggregates.

5. Maintain cells at 4°C until separated.

Protocol 4.6

Re-electrophoresis of FFE separated cells

Protocol

1. Take a suspension of cells to be electrophoresed of between 10^7 and 10^8 cells ml^{-1} and fix them in PBS containing 0.4% formaldehyde.

2. Separate the cells by FFE, employing the buffers, flow rate and electrical conditions of choice.

3. Determine which collection tubes contain cells either by cell counting, or spectrophotometric turbidity measurements at 500 or 280 nm.

4. Construct a graph of the cell separation profile.

5. Divide the cells into three or four subpopulations which contain at least 10^7 cells ml^{-1}.

6. Take two cell populations differing in electrophoretic mobility, mix them together, and resuspend in a small volume of chamber buffer (1–2 ml) so that the cell concentration is at least 10^7 cells ml^{-1}.

7. Re-electrophorese the cells under identical conditions as the original cells.

8. Construct a graph of a new cell profile. If the cells have genuinely different electrokinetic properties, two peaks coinciding with the original separation should be observed.

Note

Re-electrophoresis is best performed on the same day as the original cells.

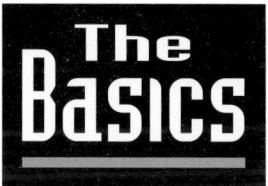

Chapter 5

Affinity separation

1. Introduction

Affinity separations include a variety of approaches to cell separation, all of which are mediated by affinity for a particular molecule. Cells are separated on the basis of differences in surface character. The basis of these separation methods is that a molecule is available that has an affinity for the surface molecule(s) that are different. The binding of these molecules is then used to 'label' the cells and by employing a variety of methods the labeled cells can be distinguished and separated. Both in principle and practice these are extremely powerful separation methods because they are based on very specific biological interactions. The affinity methods as described here can either be nonmagnetic or magnetic, with the latter the predominant and more routinely used, and are easier to perform and do not require expensive specialized equipment. Flow cytometry (also an affinity method) is described in Chapter 6.

2. Separation by nonmagnetic techniques

2.1 Affinity to fibers and solid surfaces

Cells may be separated by virtue of their affinity to fibers and solid surfaces such as plastic Petri dishes. The fibers and solid surfaces can be used in their natural state or with specific ligands coupled. Where cells have a natural affinity for fibers they can be separated by using unmodified fibers. The use of this method has largely been restricted to the separation of lymphoid cells which have a natural affinity for nylon or glass wool (Bianco *et al.*, 1970; Julius *et al.*, 1973; Trizio and Cudkowicz, 1974). The method is based on the fact that T cells do not adhere to nylon whereas other lymphoid cells such as B cells, monocytes/macrophages and neutrophils do adhere. Columns of unmodified fibers preferentially bind the B cells, monocytes/macrophages and neutrophils allowing the T cells to pass straight through. The adherent cells are removed by gently tapping the column and compressing the fiber with a small plunger. The fiber is then teased apart in the column with forceps, washed with medium and the effluent collected. The incubation and elution of cells from the fibers are performed in the presence of fetal calf serum (FCS).

However, while the nonadherent cell population consists mainly of T cells, certain T cell subsets (e.g. Fc receptor positive cells) may be specifically retained on the column. Furthermore, the purification of T cells is highly dependent on the concentration of FCS in the medium; between 5 and 10% FCS is recommended, as at lower concentrations there is increased nonspecific adherence of cells and at higher concentrations fewer adherent cells are able to bind to the fibers (Sharpe, 1988).

Cells known to be naturally adherent such as peripheral blood mono-cytes may also be isolated by adherence to solid surfaces such as plastic Petri dishes. Nonbinding cells are simply poured off while bound cells can be removed mechanically. An example is described in *Protocol 5.1*.

2.2　Affinity chromatography

Affinity chromatography of cells is basically the same as affinity chro-matography of soluble molecules such as proteins. Cells are passed through a column of beads to which an affinity ligand has been coupled. While cells with an affinity for the ligand bind to the beads and remain in the column, those cells lacking this affinity pass directly through the column. The cells bound to the column are then eluted by a change in pH, ionic concentra-tion of the column buffer or soluble ligand. A variety of different beads have been used in affinity cell separations including glass and plastic beads, cross-linked dextrans, acrylamide and agarose. In order for the cells to be able to pass rapidly through the column, the beads must be large (around 250–300 μm) in diameter.

The three major types of ligand interaction used are antibody–antigen, ligand–receptor and lectin–carbohydrate. Either molecule of these pairs can be coupled to the adsorbant and separate cells by binding to its counterpart on the cell surface. The molecules most commonly linked to the adsorbant cells are antibodies, hormones (ligand) or lectins.

Antibody coupled to the beads bind cells with a surface antigen recog-nized by the antibody. Removal of bound cells can, however, be difficult since the antibody–antigen interactions are often strong and a suitable competing agent (e.g. high concentrations of unbound antibody) may not be available. An example of affinity chromatography of cells on the basis of antibody–antigen binding is that described for the isolation of HLA-DR positive lymphocytes (*Protocol 5.2*). An alternative to direct antibody cou-pling to the adsorbant, is to use Protein A. Protein A is an immunoglobulin G (IgG) binding protein from *Staphylococcus aureus* which binds to the Fc region of IgG-type antibodies. Cells are incubated with antibody and then passed through a column of Protein A-linked adsorbant. The cells with the antibody on their surface will bind and be retained to the Protein A-linked column. These cells can be competitively eluted with IgG. This approach was applied to the separation of mouse spleen lymphocytes by Ghetie *et al.* (1978).

Where a particular cell type has a surface receptor for a ligand such as a hormone, this interaction can also be used for affinity cell separation. The purified ligand is immobilized by coupling to an adsorbant and used to retain cells on a column which have the surface receptor. The major prob-lem with this interaction is the availability of ligand (e.g. a hormone) both for coupling and elution of bound cells. However, one area where this approach has been applied is the separation of neurone and non-neurone cells as demonstrated by Dvorak *et al.* (1978).

On the other hand, column-bound lectins may be used to recognize and bind to specific carbohydrate sequences on the cell surface. The carbohydrates are usually in the form of glycoproteins and glycolipids where the carbohydrate moieties are exposed at the cell surface. Cells that have different carbohydrates on their surfaces can thus be separated by passage through a column of adsorbant to which a particular lectin is coupled. Affinity separation using lectins can only be used where a particular cell type of interest shows a specific interaction with a particular lectin and so this method is not as generally applicable as antibody–antigen interactions. However, the advantage of the lectin system is that elution of bound cells is relatively straightforward since simple monosaccharides and disaccharides compete with cells for lectin binding. An example of affinity chromatography on the basis of lectin–carbohydrate binding is that described for the separation of T and B lymphocytes by Hellström *et al.* (1984).

However, it should be noted that the most common problem with the techniques described appears to be nonspecific binding of the cells to the column material. Where this occurs, the purity of the cells separated is greatly reduced. The extent of nonspecific binding of cells is greatly dependent upon the particular cells of interest; there are very good examples of separations with certain cell types but not with most. Furthermore, many workers have been unable to obtain adequate separation, recovery or viabilities with these methods.

With the advent of magnetic beads as a solid support for antibody and the basis for (immuno)magnetic separation and enrichment, the methods described above are not currently in widespread use. However, it is worth noting the value of these techniques and the basis from which advances in immunoseparations were achieved. Indeed, there is still a niche for separation by nonmagnetic methods (Ahonen *et al.*, 1999; Murali-Krishna *et al.*, 1999; Valujskikh *et al.*, 1999).

3.   Separation by magnetic techniques

Immunomagnetic separation of cells has proven to be an effective way of obtaining pure cell subpopulations. In immunomagnetic cell separations, cells are targeted with magnetic beads coated with monoclonal antibodies specific for antigens expressed by the target cell population. The labeled cell population is then separated from the unlabeled cells by placing the sample in or passing it through a magnetic field. The cells with beads bound are retained by the magnet while the cells without beads bound are eluted or removed. Immunomagnetic beads are advantageous because they do not introduce biological products nor do they induce toxicity.

3.1 Immunomagnetic beads

A variety of magnetic particles have been produced using various substances such as starch, dextran, agarose, cellulose, albumin, methacrylate, polystyrene or styrene-divinylbenzene. Today, most, if not all, magnetic beads are paramagnetic; the beads have no permanent magnetic properties but magnetism can be induced by an applied magnetic field. The paramagnetic beads have no permanent magnetic properties after having been removed from a magnetic field; this of the utmost importance for the application of the beads in cell separation, as any remnant magnetism would severely reduce the ease of redispersion during antibody coating and cell separation.

There are several commercial suppliers of immunomagnetic beads; they include the 'MACS Microbeads' by Miltenyi and 'Dynabeads' by Dynal amongst others. While some products are available for coating with antibody by the user, others may be purchased ready coated for immediate use in separating specified cell populations. It is important to note that a procedure that works well with one particular product may not be as successful with a different product as exemplified with MACS Microbeads and Dynabeads.

3.2   Magnetic cell sorting using MACS Microbeads

With MACS, cells of interest are specifically labeled with super-paramagnetic Microbeads. After magnetic labeling, the cells are passed through a separation column (with a ferromagnetic matrix) which is placed in a strong permanent magnet. The magnetically labeled cells are retained in the column and separated from the unlabeled cells, which pass through. After removal of the column from the magnetic field, the retained fraction can be eluted. Both fractions, magnetic and nonmagnetic, are completely recovered with high purity and viability.

The small size of the MACS Microbeads (about 50 nm in diameter) distinguishes them from other beads. The beads are about one million times smaller in volume than a eukaryotic cell and comparable to the size of a virus. These magnetic microbeads are too small to be detected by light microscopy or flow cytometry, and so do not affect the light scattering of labeled cells. Thus MACS isolated cells can be immediately sorted for another parameter using flow cytometry.

However, while MACS incorporates simplicity, the technique is limited by the need for single cell suspensions. Aggregates and cell clumping can lead to blocking of the column and hinder, if not prevent, separation. In addition, it is important to remove nonviable cells and debris from the starting sample as dead cells are often nonspecifically labeled with the MicroBeads or stick to the column matrix.

3.3   Magnetic cell sorting using Dynabeads

Another development in the field of cell separation using magnetic microspheres is the availability of commercially produced immunomagnetic particles, 'Dynabeads M-450' together with a custom-built apparatus for their separation. The Dynabeads are uniform, magnetic polystyrene beads with a diameter of 4.5 µm that are supplied either uncoated or precoated with antibodies. Beads coated with antibody are used to capture target cells in a heterogeneous suspension which are recovered with a magnet, thus separating the bound target cell from the suspension. The apparatus (MPC – magnetic particle concentrator) for the separation of beads, and cells with beads bound, consists of a simple permanent magnet supported on a clamp which holds from either one to 96 test tubes containing the cell–Dynabeads mixture.

Cell separation in a tube, not a column, gives a higher yield of viable cells and allows efficient separation of cells even in viscous samples. This means that unlike column-based systems, Dynabeads can be used to isolate cells from a wide range of starting samples including whole blood, bone marrow, buffy coat, mononuclear cell suspensions and single cell suspensions prepared from tissue.

3.4   Type of separation

There are two basic strategies to isolate specific cell subpopulations: positive selection, and negative selection or depletion.

Positive selection is the capture of a desired population of cells for analysis. Target cells are magnetically labeled with the beads and subsequently isolated directly as the magnetic, positive fraction. The remaining nontarget cells are usually discarded. The isolated cells may, in many cases, be analyzed with the beads remaining attached.

Positive selection may be direct or indirect (*Figure 5.1*). In the direct technique, antibody is attached to the bead either directly onto the bead surface or through a secondary antibody prior to use as a capture reagent. This option is fast and requires very little preparation of the target cell population. An example of direct positive selection is illustrated in *Protocol 5.3*. In the indirect technique antibody is first coated onto the target cells, which are then captured with a secondary antibody-coated bead (*Protocol 5.4*). Indirect labeling is useful to amplify the magnetic label, which is particularly important if dimly expressed markers are used for magnetic separation. Another advantage of this option is the ability to use cocktails of antibodies targeting the same or multiple cells in the sample. However, a disadvantage of this approach is that cells need to be washed several times by centrifugation to remove unbound primary antibody, a procedure often resulting in loss of cell viability.

Negative selection or depletion is the removal of an unwanted population of cells from a heterogeneous mixture, leaving behind the desired population for analysis or further purification, that is, all cells are labeled apart

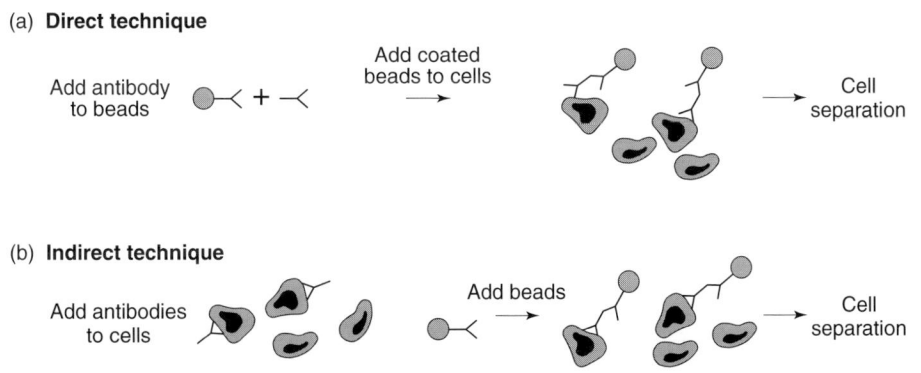

Figure 5.1

Immunomagnetic separation.

from the target cells. On magnetic separation, the magnetically labeled cells are retained in the magnetic field while the target cells are contained in the negative, nonmagnetic fraction. Selection can be direct or indirect as described above. With this approach, a depletion efficiency of 100% with purity of the captured cells (i.e. removal of unwanted cells only) is a critical factor. Unlike positive selection, viability of the labeled (depleted) cells is of less concern.

3.5   Detachment of positively selected cells

Although various analyses can be performed with the beads still bound to the cell, in many cases it is desirable or necessary to remove them. As antibody–antigen interactions are not easily resolved, except under fairly strong conditions that may be harmful to the isolated cell (e.g. acid pH), other methods are used to detach beads from cells. They include passive overnight incubation, and a combination of incubation and shear force through vigorous pipeting. Others have used limited proteolysis but this may damage surface markers and compromise further analysis.

Developments in antibody technology have provided anti-Fab antibodies which bind to the Fab region of the primary antibody and alter its affinity for antigen-producing gentle detachment. After detachment the reacting antibodies remain associated with the beads and unreacted anti-Fab may be washed away, leaving the isolated cell free of original isolating antibody.

Dynal have developed two systems for the detachment of Dynabeads from positively isolated cells: DETACHaBEAD and CELLection. DETACHaBEAD is unique to Dynal. It is a polyclonal anti-Fab antibody specific for several of the primary antibodies on Dynabeads. When DETACHaBEAD is added to the bead bound cells, it competes with antibody–antigen binding at the cell surface and releases the antibody and bead from the cells. The target cells are left viable, unstimulated and without antibody on their surface (Friedl *et al.*, 1995; Entschladen *et al.*, 1997). DETACHaBEAD is available with Dynabeads for human CD4, CD8, CD19 and CD34 cells, plus mouse CD4 cells.

CELLection Dynabeads are specifically designed for positive isolation of any cell type. Antibodies are attached to the surface of the CELLection Dynabeads via a DNA linker. This linker region provides a cleavable site to remove the beads from the cells after isolation. Cells captured by the antibody-coated beads are separated with a magnetic particle concentrator and then gently released by addition of the DNase Releasing Buffer supplied with each kit. The CELLection system is available precoated with anti-CD2 for human CD2 cell isolation, with anti-CD8 for mouse CD8 cell isolation, or BerEP4 antibody for the enrichment of epithelial tumor cells.

With regard to the Miltenyi MACS Microbeads, these are biodegradable because of their small size and their biochemical composition of iron oxide and polysaccharide, and so do not pose much of a problem. They decompose when cells are cultured. Cell function and viability are preserved. Indeed positively selected cells can be used immediately after separation for culture and subsequent studies. However, Miltenyi have also developed a system of bead detachment but have extended this to multi-sorting. For many experiments it is expedient to isolate cell subpopulations according to the expression of various antigens. MACS MultiSort technology allows the isolation of cell subpopulations according to multiple parameters, for example, CD4+CD8+ or CD34+CD38- cells. With MACS multi-parameter cell sorting, the cells of interest are magnetically labeled with MultiSort MicroBeads. Using a MACS separator, the cells of interest are positively selected according to a first parameter. Subsequently, the selected cells are incubated with MACS MultiSort Release Reagent which enzymatically removes the magnetic particles from the antibodies. In the last step, the positive cells are magnetically labeled with another antibody–MicroBead-complex and sorted according to a second cell surface marker using a MACS separator. Enzymatic removal of the MACS MultiSort MicroBeads from the cell is reported not to alter the cell surface molecules or the physiology of the cells.

Regardless of the detachment method used, the number of beads bound to the isolated cells will influence the efficiency of detachment. The number of beads used per target cell should be kept to a minimum such that the yield of released cells is increased.

3.6 Factors affecting immunomagnetic separation

Target cells

The level of antigen expression on the surface of target cells at the time of separation is important as seen with differentiating cells (Swann *et al.*, 1992). Cells with low antigen density can indeed be isolated by immunomagnetic separation but an increased number of beads may be necessary. The amount of antibody, the number of beads and the separation approach used should be optimized. As obvious as it may seem, it is important to note that after separation when the beads are bound to the cells the availability of the antigen in question will be reduced.

Antibodies

The key to successful immunomagnetic separation is the antibody of choice. Whilst polyclonal antibodies have been successfully used in the separation of cells, the use of monoclonal antibodies is favored because of their specificity. Efficient immunomagnetic separation is dependent upon the application of paramagnetic beads coated with antibody or other ligand specific to the target cells.

The choice of antibody class may influence the separation strategy used. For instance, monoclonal IgM antibodies can be coated noncovalently directly on to the surface of uncoated and nonactivated beads. Functionality of IgM does not appear to be affected by steric hindrance as a result of the nature of the pentavalent structure and size of the molecules. Though it is necessary to purify IgM (or indeed any other ligand used for direct coating) to prevent binding of other contaminating proteins or agents that may be present in the preparation. This is achieved by purification through a Sephadex G-50 column whereby IgM is collected in the void volume. An alternative to direct coating is to use beads coated with a secondary antibody which can be used to target and bind monoclonal IgM directly without the need for purification as described.

In contrast to IgM, IgG antibodies are not amenable to direct coating onto the surface of the beads. The Fab region may by incorrectly orientated with respect to the target cell and the separation affected by steric hindrance. This is overcome by the use of beads coated with a secondary antibody. The coated beads are used to specifically bind IgG onto the bead without the need for purification as described for IgM.

As for polyclonal antibodies, these are best adsorbed onto beads coated with secondary antibodies.

Monoclonal antibodies of any class can be used with the appropriate secondary antibody coated beads directly from culture supernatant since the vast majority of immunoglobulin in the system is specific antibody. However, while polyclonal sera and IgG fractions are often used directly as they tend to have a high titer of the specific antibody, affinity purified polyclonal antibodies are preferred.

The specificity of the primary antibody will without doubt determine the nature of the isolated cell type and efficiency of separation. Care must be taken to establish the antigen binding characteristics of the antibody used to eliminate undesired reactions; these can be 'specific' with the primary antibody reacting with the same or similar antigen on another cell, or 'nonspecific', for example, the binding of cells bearing surface immunoglobulin through species cross-reaction with the secondary coated antibody. These effects can usually be overcome by antibody blocking or depletion of the contaminating cell type prior to separation. Consideration should be given to the use of biotin-labeled antibodies and streptavidin-coated beads where species cross-reaction cannot be remedied.

However, as with nonmagnetic methods, other ligands (other than antibodies) can be coated onto the beads. Nonantibody ligands such as lectins can be covalently bound to the beads activated to allow chemical coupling.

The reader should refer to technical sheets or handbooks provided by the suppliers for methods on coating beads.

Other variables

While suppliers of Dynabeads and MACS Microbeads may recommend conditions such as bead to cell ratios, *et cetera*, when labeling cells, it is important to note that these conditions may not be optimal for the cell type of interest. Variables such as bead to cell ratio, volume of incubation medium, method of mixing, incubation and mixing time, and temperature become critical when high efficiencies of bead–cell interaction and subsequent separation are required (Patel and Rickwood, 1995). It was demonstrated that changing incubation conditions from the determined optimum generally resulted in poor bead binding. These findings emphasize the importance of careful optimization of every component of the separation system.

3.7 Applications

Immunomagnetic separation has become one of the most specific, reliable and fastest techniques available today for the fractionation of cells. The many different separations to which the technique has been applied are numerous and cannot be readily listed here. However, a selection is given for each of the two magnetic systems described in this chapter.

Separations routinely achieved using Dynabeads include that of platelets, reticulocytes, macrophages, spermatozoa, human dendritic cells, human endothelial cells, (non)epithelial tumor cells, lymphoma cells from bone marrow, mouse lymphocytes, *et cetera* (see Dynal Handbook). *Table 5.1* illustrates the use of Dynabeads in the separation of human peripheral blood cells. However, Dynabeads have also been used successfully in the detection of microbial pathogens in urine (Hedrum *et al.*, 1992), food and water samples (Kapperud *et al.*, 1993), blood (Seesod *et al.*, 1993) and feces (Olsvik *et al.*, 1994). Dynabeads have been used to enrich for *Salmonella* (Cudjoe *et al.*, 1994), *Escherichia coli* 0157 (Wright *et al.*, 1994), *Chlamydia trachomatis* (Hedrum *et al.*, 1992), the malaria causing parasite *Plasmodium falciparum* (Seesod *et al.*, 1993) and many more (Olsvik *et al.*, 1994).

With MACS, cells such as hematopoietic stem and progenitor cells, residual tumor cells, or antigen-specific B or T cells, NK cells, dendritic cells, fetal cells, epithelial cells, mouse lymphocytes, and apoptotic cells can be isolated and used for all kinds of analysis and functional assays. Isolation of cells according to the expression of cytoplasmic molecules or selection of live cells based on secreted proteins is also feasible. Separation of plant protoplasts is also possible (see Miltenyi handbook).

In summary, as previously stated, immunomagnetic separation is a leading technique in the separation of cells. It is one of the most specific, simplistic, reliable and fastest techniques available today for the fractionation of cells.

Table 5.1. A selection of human peripheral blood cells isolated using Dynabeads

Cell type	Type of selection	Target antigen	Efficiency yield; purity	Ref.
B lymphocytes	Positive	CD19	40–60%; > 95%	
	Negative	CD2, 14, 16	n.d.; 95%	Kim *et al.* (1992)
	Depletion	CD19, 20	>97%; n.d.	Vacca *et al.* (1991)
T lymphocytes	Positive	CD2	>90%: >99%	
	Negative	CD14, 16, 19, 56	n.d.; 97-99%	Malefyt *et al.* (1993)
T lymphocytes – CD4+	Positive	CD4	>80%; >95%	
	Negative	CD8, 14, 16, 19, 56	n.d.; >96%	Cayota *et al.* (1993)
	Depletion	CD4	>99% depletion	
T lymphocytes – CD8+	Positive	CD8	>80%; >95%	
	Depletion	CD8	>99% depletion	
T lymphocytes – antigen-specific	Positive	TCR		Kang *et al.* (1992)
NK cells	Negative	CD4, 8, 14, 19	>98%; >80%	
Monocytes	Negative	CD19, 56	n.d.; 95%	Kasinrerk *et al.* (1993)
Basophils	Negative	CD3, 4, 8, 14, 15, 19	66%; 97%	Bjerke *et al.* (1993)
Eosinophils	Negative	CD16	2–20 × 10⁷; 95%	Bach *et al.* (1990)
Neutrophils	Depletion	CD16	n.d.	Bach *et al.* (1990)
Hematopoietic	Positive	CD34	35–90%; 90%	
progenitors	Negative	CD2, 19	72%; 85%	Flø *et al.* (1991)

References

Ahonen, C.L., Gibson, S.J., Smith, R.M., Pederson, L.K., Lindh, J.M., Tomai, M.A. and Vasilakos, J.P. (1999) Dendritic cell maturation and subsequent enhanced T cell stimulation induced with the novel synthetic immune response modifier R-848 *Cell. Immunol.* **197**: 62–72.

Bach, M.K., Brashler, J.R. and Sanders, M.E. (1990) Preparation of large number of highly purified normodense human eosinophils from leukapheresis. *J. Immunol. Methods* **130**: 277–281.

Bianco, C., Patrick, R. and Nussenzweig, V. (1970) A population of lymphocytes bearing a membrane receptor for antigen-antibody-complement complexes. *J. Exp. Med.* **132**: 702–720.

Bjerke, T., Nielsen, S., Helgestad, J., Nielsen, B.W. and Schiotz, P.O. (1993) Purification of human blood basophils by negative selection using immuno-magnetic beads. *J. Immunol. Methods* **157**: 49–56.

Cayota, A., Vuillier, F., Scott-Algara, D., Feuille, V. and Dighiero, G. (1993) Differential requirements for HIV-1 replication in naive and memory CD4 T-cells from asymptomatic HIV-1 seropositive carriers and aids patients. *Clin. Exp. Immunol.* **91**: 241–248.

Cudjoe, K.S., Krona, R. and Olsen, E. (1994) IMS: A new selective enrichment technique for detection of Salmonella in foods. *Int. J. Food Microbiol.* **23**: 159–165.

Dvorak, D. J., Gipps, E. and Kidson, C. (1978) Isolation of specific neurones by affinity methods. *Nature* **271**: 564–566.

Entschladen, F., Niggemann, B., Zanker, K.S. and Friedl, P. (1997) Differential requirement of protein tyrosine kinases and protein kinase C in the regulation of T cell locomotion in three-dimensional collagen matrices. *J. Immunol.* **159**: 3203–3210.

Flø, R.W., Næss, A., Lund-Johansen, F., Mæhle, B, Sjursen, H., Lehmann, V. and Solberg, C. (1991) Negative selection of human monocytes using magnetic particles covered by anti-lymphocyte antibodies. *J. Immunol. Methods* **137**: 89–94.

Friedl, P., Noble, P.B. and Zanker, K.S. (1995) T lymphocyte locomotion in a three-dimensional collagen matrix. *J. Immunol.* **154**: 4973–4985.

Ghetie, V., Mota, G. and Sjöquist, J. (1978) Separation of cells by affinity chromatography on SpA-Sepharose 6MB. *J. Immunol. Methods* **21**: 133–141.

Hedrum, A., Lundeberg, J., Påhlson, C., Uhlén, M. (1992) Immunomagnetic recovery of *Chlamydia trachomatis* from urine with subsequent colorimetric DNA detection. *PCR Meth. Appl.* **2**: 167–171.

Hellström, U., Hammarström, M.-L., Hammarström, S. and Perlmann, P. (1984) Fractionation of human lymphocytes on *Helix pomatia* A hemagglutinin-Sepharose and wheat germ agglutinin-Sepharose. In *Methods in Enzymology*, Vol. 108 (eds G. Di Sabato, J. J. Langone and H. van Vunakis). Academic Press, New York, pp. 153–168.

Julius, M.H., Simpson, E. and Herzenberg, L.A. (1973) A rapid method for the isolation of functional thymus-derived murine lymphocytes. *Eur. J. Immunol.* **3**: 645–649.

Kang, S.-M., Tran, A.-C., Grilli, M. and Lenardo, M.J. (1992) NF-kappa-β subunit regulation in nontransformed CD4+ lymphocytes. *Science* **256**: 1452–1456.

Kapperud, G., Vardund, T., Skjerve, E., Hornes, E., Michaelsen, T.E. (1993) Detection of *Yersinia enterocolitica* in foods and water by immunomagnetic separation, nested polymerase chain reactions, and colorimetric detection of amplified DNA. *Appl. Env. Microbiol.* **59**: 2938–2944.

Kasinrerk, W., Baumruker, T., Majdic, O., Knapp, W. and Stockinger, H. (1993) CD1 molecule expression on human monocytes induced by granulocyte-macrophage colony-stimulating factor. *J. Immunol.* **150**: 579–584.

Kim, K.-M., Ishigami, T., Hata, D., Higaki, Y., Morita, M., Yamaoka, K., Mayumi, M. and Mikawa, H. (1992) Anti-IgM but not anti-IgD antibodies inhibit cell division of normal human mature B-cells. *J. Immunol.* **148**: 29–34.

Malefyt, R., Yssl, H. and de Vries, J.E. (1993) Direct effects of IL-10 on subsets of human CD4⁺ T-cell clones and resting T-cells specific-inhibition of IL-2 production and proliferation. *J. Immunol.* **150:** 4754–4765.

Murali-Krishna, K., Lau, L.L., Sambhara, S., Lemonnier, F., Altmann, J. and Ahmed, R. (1999) Persistence of memory CD8 T cells in MHC Class I-deficient mice. *Science* **286:** 1377–1381.

Olsvik, Ø, Popovic, T., Skjerve, E., Cudjoe, K.S., Hornes, E., Ugelstad, J. and Uhlén, M. (1994) Magnetic separation techniques in diagnostic microbiology. *Clin. Microbiol. Rev.* **7:** 43–54.

Patel, D. and Rickwood D. (1995) Optimization of conditions for specific binding of antibody-coated beads to cells. *J. Immunol. Methods* **184:** 71–80.

Seesod, N., Lundeberg, J., Hedrum, A., Åslund, L., Holder, A., Thaithong, S. and Uhlén, M. (1993) Immunomagnetic purification to facilitate DNA diagnosis of *Plasmodium falciparum. J. Clin. Microbiol.* **31:** 2715–2719.

Sharpe, P.T. (1988) *Methods of Cell Separation.* Elsevier, Amsterdam.

Swann, I.D., Dealtry, G.B. and Rickwood, D. (1992) Differentiation-related changes in quantitative binding of immunomagnetic beads. *J. Immunol. Methods* **152:** 245–251.

Trizio, D. and Cudkowicz, G. (1974) Separation of T and B lymphocytes by nylon wool columns: evaluation of efficacy by functional assays *in vivo. J. Immunol.* **113:** 1093–1097.

Vacca, A., Di Stefano, R., Frassanito, A., Iodice, G. and Dammacco, F. (1991) A disturbance of the IL-2/IL-2 receptor system parallels the activity of multiple-myeloma. *Clin. Exp. Immunol.* **84:** 429–434.

Valujskikh, A., Matesic, D. and Heeger, P.S. (1999) Characterization and manipulation of T cell immunity to skin grafts expressing a transgenic minor antigen. *Transplantation* **68:** 1029–1036.

Wright, D.J., Chapman, P.A. and Siddons, C.A. (1994) Immunomagnetic separation as a sensitive method for isolating *Escherichia coli* 0157 from food samples. *Epidemiol. Infect.* **113:** 31–39.

Bioscience Products, *Biomagnetic Techniques in Molecular Biology, and Cell Separation* handbooks. Dynal AS, Oslo, Norway.

Magnetic Cell Sorting and Separation of Biomolecules handbook. Miltenyi Biotec, Germany.

Protocol 5.1

Isolation of monocytes by adherence to solid surfaces

Equipment

Plastic Petri dishes

Humidified box/CO_2 incubator

Pipets

Rubber 'policeman'

Bench-top centrifuge

Centrifuge tubes

Reagents

McCoys culture medium

FCS

Serum-free RPMI

Protocol

1. Incubate Petri dish with 1 ml FCS for 45 min at 37°C.

2. Aspirate FCS. Add 2 ml leukocytes at 5×10^6 ml^{-1} isolated from whole blood to Petri dish.

3. Incubate for 60 min at 37°C.

4. Pour off supernatant and nonadherent cells.

5. Wash off remaining nonadherent cells from Petri dish with McCoys medium containing 10% FCS at 37°C.

6. Release bound monocytes by incubating Petri dish with serum-free RPMI for 15 min at 22°C. Repeat twice. Removal of bound cells is enhanced by scraping the Petri dish with a rubber 'policeman'.

7. Collect monocytes from washings by low-speed centrifugation.

Note

Use aseptic techniques to maintain sterility. Perform procedure in a laminar flow-hood if necessary.

Protocol 5.2

Isolation of HLA-DR positive lymphocytes using antibody–antigen binding

Equipment

Plastic column

End-over-end mixer

Bench-top centrifuge

Centrifuge tubes

Vortex mixer

Reagents

CNBr-activated Sepharose 4B

Hydrochloric acid

Bicarbonate buffer: 0.1 M NaHCO$_3$, 0.5 M NaCl pH 7.7

Monoclonal antibody specific for HLA-DR, e.g. ATCC L243

Ethanolamine

Acetate buffer: 0.1 M sodium acetate, 0.5 M NaCl pH 4.0

Phosphate-buffered saline (PBS)

Sodium azide

FCS

40% Percoll

Protocol

Preparation of antibody column

1. Place 1 g CNBr-activated Sepharose 4B in a 12 ml plastic column.

2. Wash column with 20 ml 1 mM HCl.

3. Wash column with 20 ml bicarbonate buffer.

4. Cease flow-through and add 10 ml bicarbonate buffer to column.

5. Add 6 mg antibody in 1 ml bicarbonate buffer to column.

6. Seal column. Rotate column on end-over-end mixer slowly for 2 h at 22°C.

7. Wash column with 250 ml bicarbonate buffer.

8. Add 10 ml ethanolamine and rotate as in step 6.

9. Wash column as in step 7 followed by acetate buffer. Repeat washes.

10. Wash column with 50 ml PBS containing 0.01% sodium azide.

11. Store column at 4°C.

Isolation of HLA-DR positive lymphocytes

1. Suspend isolated lymphocytes (at a maximum of 1×10^7 ml^{-1}) in 5 ml PBS containing 20% FCS.

2. Add lymphocyte suspension to column, seal, and incubate for 20 min at 20°C.

3. Incubate for 20 min at 4°C.

4. Remove Sepharose and cell suspension from column and layer on to 10 ml 40% Percoll. Centrifuge at 700 *g* for 20 min at 20°C.

5. Harvest HLA-DR positive cells bound to the Sepharose from the interface.

6. Wash cells in 5 ml PBS and pellet at 400 *g* for 10 min.

7. Vortex in 5 ml 40% Percoll and centrifuge at 700 *g* for 20 min to remove lymphocytes from Sepharose.

8. Recover HLA-DR positive lymphocytes from layer above Percoll.

Note

Use aseptic techniques to maintain sterility.

Protocol 5.3

Direct positive selection of CD4$^+$ T cells from whole blood

Equipment

Dynabeads M-450 CD4

Magnetic particle concentrator

Pipets

Mixer

10-ml plastic tissue culture grade round-bottomed tubes

Reagents

2 ml EDTA or ACD anticoagulated blood

PBS containing 0.6% sodium citrate

PBS containing 1% FCS or BSA

Culture media or Tris balanced salt solution (TBSS) pH 7.4: 4 g NaCl, 0.2 g KCl, 0.1 g MgSO$_4$.7H$_2$O, 29.25 mg Tris

Protocol

Preparation of Dynabeads M-450 CD4

1. Calculate the volume of Dynabeads required for the separation in question.

2. Resuspend beads. Pipet out desired amount of beads into a 10-ml tube.

3. Place the tube on a magnetic particle concentrator for 1 min. Where the volume is small it may be necessary to make up to a workable volume with PBS containing FCS.

4. Aspirate the supernatant. Resuspend the beads in PBS containing FCS and return to magnet. Aspirate supernatant. Resuspend beads to original volume with PBS containing FCS.

Isolation of cells

1. Collect 5 ml blood in a standard ACD blood collecting tube.

2. Cool blood, buffers and Dynabeads to 4°C.

3. Add the blood to the Dynabeads directly in the 10-ml tube.

4. Mix gently for 30–60 min by tilting and rotation.

5. Add 5 ml PBS pH 7.4 containing 0.6% sodium citrate.

6. Isolate the rosetted cells by placing the tube in the magnetic particle concentrator for 2–3 min.

7. Discard the supernatant while the rosetted cells are attracted to the wall of the tube by the magnet.

8. Wash the isolated cells. First remove the tube from the magnet. Resuspend the rosetted cells in 5 ml PBS pH 7.4 containing 0.6% sodium citrate. Replace the tube in the magnetic particle concentrator for a minimum of 2 min to collect the rosetted cells. Discard the supernatant and resuspend the rosetted cells in 5 ml PBS containing BSA pH 7.4 without sodium citrate. Repeat washing 2–3 times as described.

9. Resuspend rosetted cells in the desired volume of culture media or TBSS.

Notes

If the volume for final resuspension of the rosetted cells is small (<0.5 ml), resuspend cells in 0.5–1.0 ml and place in the concentrator. Once rosetted cells are attracted to the magnet slowly remove the tube vertically and in doing so concentrate the cells in a pellet. Alternatively, after resuspension in the larger volume, transfer to a microcentrifuge tube and concentrate using a magnetic particle concentrator appropriate for such tubes. Resuspend cells in desired volume.

In step 8 of 'Isolation of cells' resuspend cells by adding the buffer into the tube on the opposite side of the line of cells to minimize shear forces etc. from pipeting. Gentle inversion of the tube several times should allow the cells to resuspend completely into the buffer. Vigorous shaking should be avoided.

Use aseptic techniques to maintain sterility.

Protocol 5.4

Preparation of antibody-coated cells for use in indirect positive selection

Equipment

10-ml plastic round-bottomed tissue culture grade tubes

Low-speed centrifuge

Pipets

Reagents

PBS at pH 7.4

Tissue culture media; Hank's balanced salt solution (HBSS) pH 7.4 or similar

Antibody

Protocol

1. Incubate the cell sample with sufficient antibody at 4°C for 30 min.

2. Harvest the antibody-coated cells by centrifugation at 800 **g** for 10 min and discard the supernatant.

3. Resuspend the cells in HBSS and wash by centrifugation a further two times to remove all unbound antibody.

4. Resuspend the cells in HBSS or similar, and adjust volume to allow the use of $1–2 \times 10^7$ Dynabeads ml^{-1} at a minimum bead:target cell ratio of 4:1.

5. Isolate the target cells coated with specific antibody with secondary coated immunomagnetic beads, otherwise apply the same technical considerations for direct isolation.

Notes

The amount of antibody used depends on the number of target cells, and the antigen density. Saturating amounts are recommended.

Use aseptic techniques to maintain sterility.

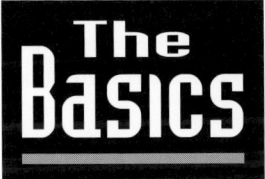

Chapter 6

Flow cytometry

1. Introduction

Flow cytometry or sorting is a process in which measurements of physical and/or chemical characteristics of cells are made while cells pass in a single file, through the measuring apparatus in a liquid stream. Cells in a liquid medium flow individually at high speed through an intense beam of light usually from a laser. As each individual cell passes through the beam, optical and electrical signals are produced, which are accurately measured. The signal may represent fluorescence, light scatter or light absorbance. Individual cells exhibiting particular properties, for example, a particular level of fluorescence emission, can be selected (*Figure 6.1*). The important feature of flow cytometry is that measurements are made separately on each particle within the suspension and not just as average values for the whole

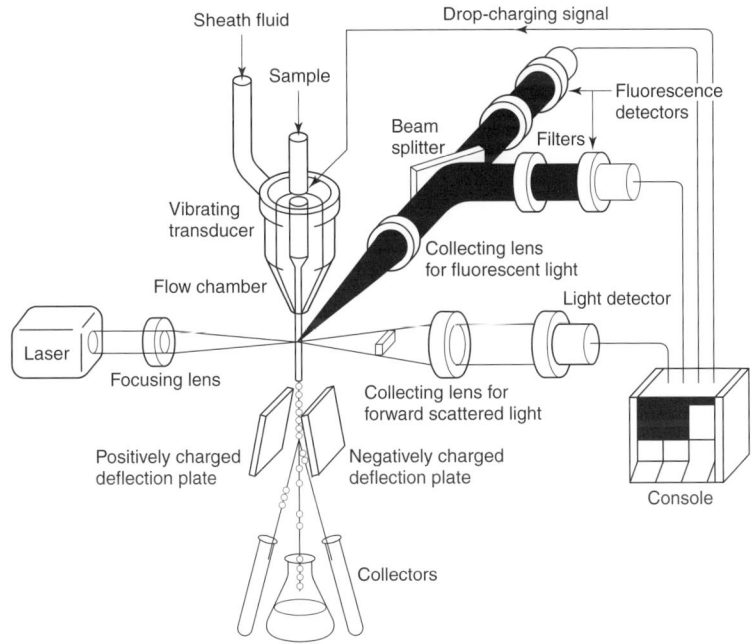

Figure 6.1

Flow cytometry.

population. The technique enables subpopulations of cells or particles to be separated from the sample suspension with a high degree of purity. The purified fractions can be used for morphological examination or in functional or other assays.

Flow cytometry is without question one of the most powerful techniques of cell separation currently available. Much of current use of this technique has been for separating cells that have surface antigens for a specific antibody. By either conjugating a fluorescent molecule to the antibody or by using a fluorescent second antibody, the cells can be separated on the basis of the fluorescence emitted.

Flow cytometry is achieved via automated cell sorters, often referred to as fluorescence activated cell sorters or FACS. By far the most extensive use of flow sorting in cell separation is the separation of cells specifically labeled with a fluorescent molecule or tag, hence the common name of fluorescent activated cell sorting. The same apparatus can however also be used to separate cells of different sizes based on their light scattering properties.

It is beyond the aim of this chapter to present detailed information of flow sorting with specific instruments as each has slightly different modes of operation. This chapter is limited to the principle of flow sorting and examples of the kind of separations that can be obtained.

2.   The flow cytometer – instrumentation

The basic flow cytometer consists of a light source, a flow chamber, optics to focus light of different wavelengths on to the detectors, and signal detection and processing units.

2.1   Light source

In most flow cytometers, the light source is an argon-ion laser tuned to produce blue light (488 nm). Most cell sorters can accommodate a second laser such that cells may be excited at two different wavelengths. Lasers can be either small or large. Small lasers are air-cooled and are usually of a fixed emission at 488 nm. Large lasers are water-cooled and can be tuned to other wavelengths, particularly in the UV at 360–380 nm. Argon-ion lasers tuned to 488 nm were initially chosen as this wavelength could be used to excite fluorescein – a fluorochrome widely used as a label or tag (conjugated to an antibody). However, many dyes have been produced that can also be excited by blue light; such developments have meant that with a single laser, many immunofluorescent signals can be observed (*Table 6.1*). Dyes that require excitation in the UV include Hoechst 33342 and 33258 that label DNA, and indo-1 used to measure intracellular calcium ion. A selection of fluorophores is given in *Table 1.4*, Chapter 1. Some instruments employ mercury arc lamps as opposed to argon-ion lasers. Though they may be useful as an inexpensive source of light, sensitivity is reduced. Small air-cooled lasers may also be helium–neon (emission at 544 or 633 nm) and helium–cadmium (325 nm).

2.2   Flow chamber

The purpose of the flow chamber is to deliver cells singly to a specific point at which the light source is focused (the detection point). The sample is

Table 6.1. Fluorochromes that can be excited by blue light at 488 nm

Dyes	Used to label	Excitation max. (nm)	Emission max. (nm)[a]	Color of emitted light
Fluorescein	Protein	495	520	Green
Peridinin chlorophyll conjugate (perCP)	Protein	490	677	Deep red
R-phycoerythrin	Protein	564, 495	576	Orange
Phycoerythrin-cyanine-5 conjugate (Cy-chrome)	Protein	490	670	Deep red
Phycoerythrin-Texas Red conjugate (ECD)	Protein	495	620	Red
Propidium iodide	DNA, RNA	495, 342	639	Red

[a]Wavelength of absorption and emission may depend on the environment of the fluorochrome.

injected into the center of a stream of liquid (sheath fluid). The chamber is designed such that the sheath fluid focuses the sample delivering the cells to the point of detection with an accuracy of ±1 µm or better. Three types of flow chamber are in general use (*Figure 6.2*). The first consists of a quartz cuvette placed at right angles to the laser beam. The cross-section of the

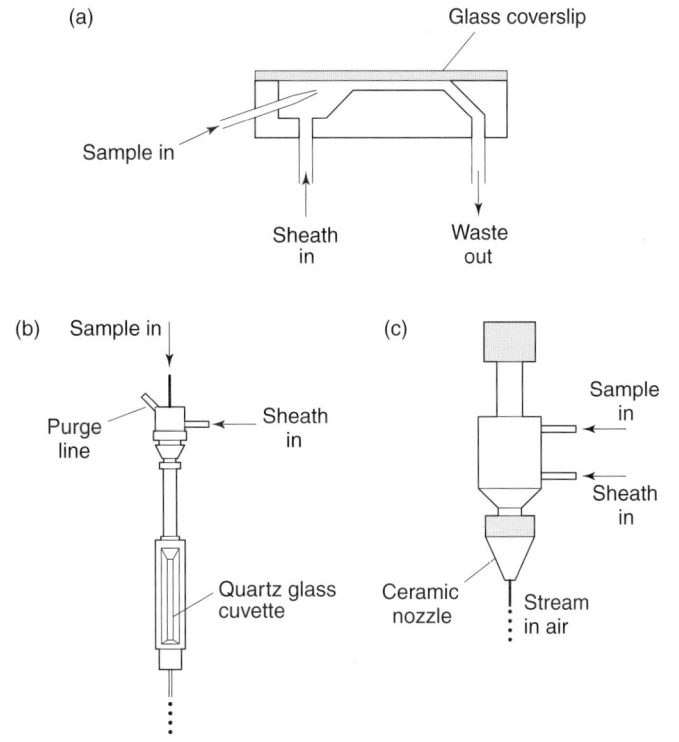

Figure 6.2

Types of flow-chamber. From Omerod (1994) Flow Cytometry: A Practical Approach, *2nd edn, with permission from Oxford University Press.*

channel is about 250 μm. Cells travel through the cuvette at about 1 m s^{-1}. Both fluorescence and light scatter can be measured over a wide angle at right angles to the focused light source; though light scatter measured in the forward direction requires an obscuration bar to block the main laser beam. The second, a frequently used design, employs stream-in-air or jet-in-air. The sheath fluid containing the focused sample stream emerges in to the air from a narrow nozzle or outlet just below which the laser beam is focused. The outlet is narrower in diameter than the flow chamber. The cells accelerate as they emerge into the air traveling at about 10 m s^{-1}. Again, fluorescence and light scatter are measured over a wide angle at right angles to the laser beam; however, two obscuration bars are necessary for measuring light scatter. In the third design, the sheath fluid and sample are forced through a channel cut in a block chamber. Fluorescence is measured along the same optical path as the excitation light. However, light scatter is difficult to measure in this design. The ultimate sensitivity of the cytometer depends upon the type of flow chamber used, with jet-in-air systems being less sensitive than the cuvette system. As indicated, the third design is the least sensitive.

2.3   Optical components

The laser beam is focused onto the sample stream using a lens yielding a beam cross-section of about 50 μm. Beams can be wide and flat or circular in cross-section depending on the lenses used. Beams that are wide and flat are used with the cuvette flow chambers, while the circular cross-section beams are used with the stream-in-air systems.

Subsequent light collection from cells is achieved by the collection lens. A high numerical aperture is used in order to collect as much of the fluorescence as possible. A simple long-working distance lens is sufficient for collection of forward-scattered light.

2.4   Light scatter

As the cells pass through the laser beam, light is scattered. The light scattered at angles of less than 2° (small angle scatter) is proportional to cell size for spherical cells. Light is also scattered at 90°, which is related to the cellular contents. A cell with a rough surface membrane will scatter more intensely at 90° than a cell with a smoother membrane. A cell with many complex intracellular organelles (mitochondria, etc.) will give a larger side-scatter signal than a cell with fewer intracellular organelles. The combination of these independent values provides a great deal of information concerning cell size and morphology. Side-scatter and forward scatter together allow reliable identification of distinct populations such as platelets, red blood cells, mononuclear cells and polymorphonuclear cells in a mixture. The scatter signals received are analyzed and displayed as a dot plot or histogram (*Figure 6.3*). Each dot represents a value of the light scatter by a single cell. The scatter signals received and processed can be used as a basis for cell sorting by selecting for droplets containing one cell population to be charged positive, another population to be charged negative leaving the third uncharged.

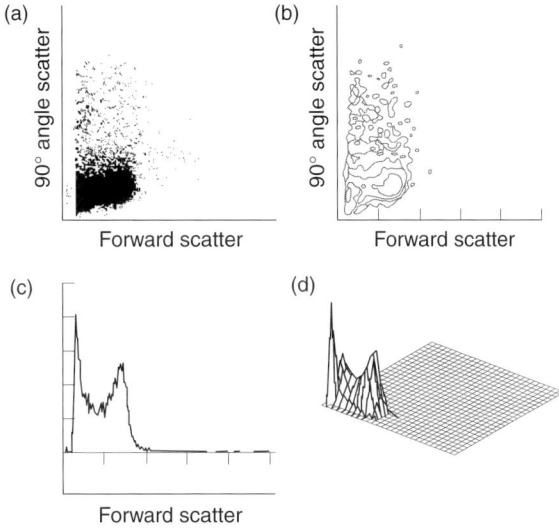

Figure 6.3

Signal output displays from a flow cytometer. (a) dot plot, (b) contour plot, (c) histogram, and (d) net or 3D plot.

2.5   Signal detection and processing

Scatter and fluorescence parameters are all forms of light that have to be collected and quantitated. Signal detection is achieved using a photodiode (for measuring forward light scatter) and photomultiplier tubes (PMT) (for measuring fluorescence scatter). The PMT is used on all cytometers to measure what can be very dim fluorescence and side scatter signals, by capturing photons of light on a light sensitive surface that elicits an electron cascade. In contrast, a photodiode is used for forward scatter analysis as this signal is usually of the highest intensity so a 'less sensitive' semi-conductor can be used. Light is collected over a narrow angle, usually in the range 2–20° in line with the illuminating beam. The signal output from the detectors is amplified and then processed. The processed signal is then converted from analogue to digital form and then transferred to computer. The signal outputs from the flow sorter can be presented in four ways (*Figure 6.3*). Each of the plots illustrates the same data.

2.6   Fluorescence

When a cell labeled with a fluorochrome passes through the beam, it absorbs light at the incident wavelength and emits the light at a longer wavelength. The light is emitted throughout 360° but is collected through a detector system at 90° to the laser beam. If several different fluorochromes are used, each emits a different wavelength and so is detected separately. The resulting photons of light received by the detectors are converted by photomultiplier tubes into electrical signals that are processed by the sorter into a digital signal. The digital signals are displayed as in *Figure*

6.3. Each dot or point on a plot display is the fluorescence signal emitted by a single cell.

2.7 Gating

At least five different measurements can be made simultaneously on each individual cell in a stream, for example, size, cell contents and fluorescent emission at several different wavelengths (termed multiparametric analysis). A particular subpopulation of cells with certain characteristics can be selected to be sorted by selecting upper and lower limits of the particular parameter(s) – termed gating. Once limits are selected, the information is relayed via the computer to the droplet charger, which conveys an electrical charge to each of the droplets containing the selected cells that are subsequently deflected from the main stream by the charged plates in a collecting vessel.

3. Types of flow sorting

3.1 Cell sorting by droplet formation

By far the commonest method of separating cells by flow cytometry is electrostatic deflection of charged droplets. The sheath fluid, buffered saline, travels through the flow chamber. The flow chamber is vibrated vertically causing the pressurized liquid stream emerging from the exit nozzle to break up into regularly spaced droplets; the applied (constant) vibration is produced by mounting the flow chamber in a piezoelectric transducer to which a regular voltage is applied (this vibration is referred to as a transducer wave). The flow chamber is charged at the moment a cell of interest is inside the droplet currently being formed. The stream of droplets then passes through an electrostatic field formed between a pair of high-voltage plates. The charged droplets are attracted to the opposite pole and collected together with the cell contained therein. The charged droplets become separated from the uncharged or oppositely charged droplets. As is it possible to apply either a negative or a positive charge to a droplet, cells can be sorted to the left or to the right of the undeflected stream (*Figures 6.1* and *6.4*). Three sorted cell populations can be collected at the same time for further study. About 10 000 cells s^{-1} is generally the maximum achievable flow-rate. Further aspects of cell sorting by droplet deflection are discussed below.

3.2 Cell sorting by deflection of the sample stream

Although most flow cytometry is by electrostatic deflection of charged droplets, some flow cytometers sort cells by deflection of the sample stream. Some instruments have a flow chamber based on a microscope stage, while others have a vertical quartz flow chamber with a closed fluidic system. In the former, the fluid stream flows horizontally through a channel that separates after the observation point. Unsorted cells travel along one arm while a piezoelectric fluidic valve deflects the sorted cells along the other arm. This approach can be used for sorting large cells, such as protoplasts, or clusters of cells, as the limitations of size imposed in the electrostatic sorters is avoided. The maximum achievable sort rate is 1000 cells s^{-1}. In sorters with

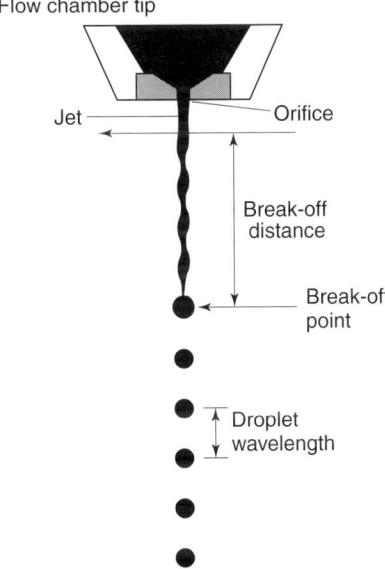

Figure 6.4

Schematic diagram showing droplet formation. From Omerod M.G. (1994) Flow Cytometry: A Practical Approach, *2nd edn, with permission from Oxford University Press.*

a vertical quartz flow chamber, a piezoelectric device deflects a small collector in to the center of the sample stream to gather a cell selected for sorting. The collector will sit on the periphery of the sample stream so that it collects sheath fluid even when a cell is not being sorted. The position of the deflector is thus critical. The maximum achievable sort rate is 300 cells s^{-1}. While sort rates are comparatively low, only one subpopulation is sorted, and sorted cells are heavily diluted, these sorters are simple to operate and can be fully enclosed allowing biological hazardous samples to be sorted.

4.   Factors affecting cell sorting

The stability of the cell sorter is affected by the viscosity of the water or fluid that is temperature dependent. Any change in viscosity will alter the speed of the jet and hence the distance between the nozzle of the flow chamber and the exit point at which a droplet is formed. Hence it is advisable that constant temperature is maintained. Others include the presence of a draught, or dirt in the flow chamber orifice. All will influence the position of the break-off point of the droplets.

The droplet break-off point is also governed by the amplitude of the transducer wave. For example, in a stream-in-air system, vibration of the stream will affect the light scattered at the stream–air interface. The transducer amplitude used is a trade-off between the requisite for having a large vibration to yield stable droplets, the need to minimize any effect on signal detection, and the need to minimize the distance between the detection and break-off points. Furthermore, the cells themselves can affect droplet formation. When a cell is within or close to the orifice when a droplet is formed, or passes through the orifice, this disturbance can either alter the timing or break-off point, respectively.

Cell sorting is accomplished only if selected cells are contained within a charged droplet. The droplets are charged by the application of a charging pulse during formation. To ensure that the flow chamber and hence droplets are charged at the correct moment, it is necessary to determine the time taken for a cell to travel from the laser beam (detection point) to the droplet break-off point. Accurate deflection is only achieved when the whole of the charge pulse is applied to the relevant droplet; a partial charge on a neighboring droplet must be avoided.

Conditions for droplet formation and charge may be changed if necessary, protocols for which are set out in the instruction manual specific to the model and type of flow cytometer. The following protocols (*Protocols 6.1 and 6.2*) are given as guides; refer to manufacturer's instruction manual for exact protocols.

Sample preparation can also hinder separation. Often during sorting, two cells may arrive close to one another at the detection point. As a result, the cells are not recognized as being separate. This can be minimized by ensuring that the number of clumped cells is reduced to a minimum during sample preparation. Further steps can be taken by gating on light scatter to exclude larger particles. It is also important to remove any debris from the sample before application to the sorter. Any debris that is too small to be detected by light scatter will not be recognized and will contaminate the sorted sample. A suspension of single cells is essential to successful flow sorting. The sample should contain as little and as few dead cells and clumps as possible. Dead cells and debris can be removed by sedimentation through a density gradient (Chapter 2). If sorting cells from peripheral blood, it is advisable to remove contaminating erythrocytes by centrifugation in a density gradient. Differential lysis may also be used to remove erythrocytes.

During sample preparation, there may also be a temptation to increase the amount of fluorescence by using higher concentrations of reagent or in the case of immunofluorescence by using reagents with a higher fluorochrome to protein ratio. This should be avoided as at high concentrations of dye the excitation energy may be dissipated as light emitted from one fluorescent molecule can be quenched by a neighboring molecule. Furthermore, fluorophores such as FITC are highly charged molecules and can lead to increased nonspecific binding of immunoglobulin if present at too great a concentration in the conjugate.

In summary, obtaining a good immunophenotyping result depends on accurate set-up of the flow sorter, selecting the correct sample, choosing the correct panel of monoclonal antibodies and fluorescent conjugates (should fluorescence be the method of selection), performing reliable staining techniques on the bench, followed by acquisition of data, its analysis, and inevitably interpretation of results.

5.   Separation – purity, yield and sterility

Flow cytometry is used to define, enrich for and to enumerate subpopulations of cells. The purity of the sorted sample may be measured by reanalyzing the sorted cells in the flow cytometer. Before doing so, the sample delivery system should be flushed through thoroughly as there may be unsorted cells still remaining in the sample delivery line. On reanalysis, the sorted cells may show slightly weakened immunofluorescence, a result of bleaching as they pass through the laser beam. Both 'purity' and yield are recorded by the computer. It is also wise to compare the yield of cells recorded by the computer to that determined experimentally to see whether the yields concur (*Protocol 6.3*). Occasionally, low yields may become a problem. Reasons for low yields may include setting incorrect drop delay measurements and/or the wrong sort mode for the sample type. Other factors include low cell content in the unsorted fraction, poor quality side streams, and even static in the sort chamber/collection tubes. These are remedied by enriching the pre-sort, checking settings or blockages, and by connecting a wire from the collection tubes to a metal surface on the cytometer to earth. As with regard to sterility, because the droplets are deflected in air, sterile sorting is not strictly possible without enclosing the whole flow chamber assembly in a sterile hood. However, with various precautions, it is possible to sort cells that can be maintained in culture for 1–2 weeks without growth of contaminants (*Protocol 6.4*).

6. Applications

The use of flow cytometers for cell sorting is widespread. Applications range from the separation of large numbers of cells for functional studies or chromosomes for preparing gene libraries to the direct cloning of single rare transfected or hybridoma cells.

Flow cytometry is an extremely powerful technique and has been used extensively in leucocyte and bone marrow immunophenotyping (Anderson *et al.*, 1984; Azzolina *et al.*, 1990; Gross *et al.*, 1995; Hoang *et al.*, 1983; Loken and Lanier, 1984; Nicola *et al.*, 1981; Sartor and Bradstock, 1994). By examining large numbers of cells, flow cytometry can give quantitative data on the percentage of cells bearing different molecules, such as surface immunoglobulin, which characterizes B cells, the T-cell receptor-associated molecules known as CD3, and the CD4 and CD8 co-receptor proteins that distinguish the major T-cell subsets. Likewise, FACS analysis has been instrumental in defining stages in the early development of B and T cells. FACS analysis has been applied to a broad range of problems in immunology; indeed, it has played a vital role in the early identification of AIDS as a disease in which T cells bearing CD4 are depleted selectively.

Indeed, the first fluorescence-activated cell sorters were primarily used in immunological applications to sort and characterize lymphocytes. However, flow sorters have since been used to separate or sort a wide variety of types of cell. In fact, any cell that can be prepared as a suspension of single cells may be analyzed and sorted by flow cytometry. As previously stated, the cells to be separated are most commonly selected by labeling the cells with fluorescent antibodies to cell surface antigens. By either coupling a fluorescent molecule direct to the antibody or by using a fluorescent second antibody, the cells are separated on the basis of the fluorescence emitted. However, cell sorting can be used to sort cells using any suitable parameter. For example, Clara cells from rat lungs have been sorted on their increased content of glutathione (Davies *et al.*, 1990). Furthermore, as seen with immunohistochemistry (Chapter 1, Section 6.7), if a suitable substrate is available, cells can be analyzed and sorted according to an enzyme activity. For example, the detection of the presence of the *Escherichia coli* β-D-galactosidase gene (*lacZ*) in mammalian cells (Fiering *et al.*, 1991). Alternatively, the DNA content of a cell can be measured by staining the DNA with a dye that binds to the nucleic acid stoichiometrically and whose fluorescence is enhanced upon binding. Measurement of the DNA content of a cell provides a picture of the cell cycle and is an important tool in the study of action of cytotoxic drugs. For instance, in clinical samples, DNA content gives the DNA ploidy of a tumor. An estimation of the S phase fraction is a measure of the proliferative state of the tumor.

Flow cytometry has become a standard method of analysis particularly in immunology and in clinical laboratories. However, the technique is not limited to eukaryotic cells, indeed, flow cytometry can be used for the rapid analysis of bacterial populations and provides information difficult to obtain by other techniques. Assessment of microbial viability is a major requirement in several areas including public health, biotechnology, food technology, the water industry and the pharmaceutical industry. One indicator of viability is the ability of the cell membrane to exclude dyes and retain cell contents. Other approaches include the uptake of either fluorescent probes such as oxonol (Carter *et al.*, 1993; Kaprelyants and Kell, 1992), or uncharged nonfluorescent lipophilic fluorogenic substrates such as fluorescein esters (Diaper and Edwards, 1994; Jepras *et al.*, 1995). The use of flow cytometry and appropriate viability probes allow the rapid assessment of antibiotic activity and can provide an insight into their mode of action. These are just some examples of flow cytometry and its immense capability.

In brief, one of the advantages of flow cytometry is the high purity that can be achieved (usually >95%). Second, small subpopulations can be selected for (1% or fewer of the starting cell suspension), and third, several parameters can be used to select the cells for sorting. The technique can be used to define, enrich for, and to enumerate accurately subpopulations. Flow cytometers can measure several parameters on single cells at rates of hundreds to thousands of cells per second. However, the major problem experienced by laboratories is the expense of, and in turn, the access to a flow cytometer. Another disadvantage of flow sorting is the low throughout of cells compared to other methods. About 10 000 cells s^{-1} is generally the maximum achievable flow-rate. When the required throughput is large, mechanical means of separating cells are preferable (Chapters 2 and 5), if not only as a pre-purification step.

Further reading

Ormerod, M.G. (1994) *Flow Cytometry*. RMS Handbook No. 29. BIOS Scientific Publishers, Oxford.

Pinkel, D. and Stovel, R. (1985) In *Flow Cytometry Instrumentation and Data Analysis* (eds M.A. Van Dilla, P.N. Dean, O.D. Laerum and M.R. Melamed). Academic Press, Orlando, pp. 77–128.

References

Anderson, K.C., Bates, M.P., Slaughenhoupt, B.L., Pinkus, G.S., Schlossman, S.F. and Nadler, L.M. (1984) Expression of human B cell-associated antigens on leukemias and lymphomas: a model of human B cell differentiation. *Blood* **63**: 1424–1433.

Azzolina, L.S., Stevanoni, G., Tommasi, M. and Tridente, G. (1990) Phenotypic analysis of human peripheral blood lymphocytes by automatic sampling flow cytometry after stimulation with mitogens or allogeneic cells. *Res. Clinic Laboratory* **20**: 209–216.

Carter, E.A., Paul, F.E. and Hunter, P.A. (1993) Cytometric evaluation of antifungal agents. In: *Flow Cytometry in Microbiology* (ed. D. Lloyd). Springer-Verlag, London, pp. 111–120.

Davies, R., Cain, K., Edwards, R.E., Snowden, R.T., Legg, R.F. and Neal, G.E. (1990) The preparation of highly enriched fractions of binucleated rat hepatocytes by centrifugal elutriation and flow cytometry. *Anal. Biochem.* **190**: 266–270.

Diaper, J.P. and Edwards, C. (1994) The use of fluorogenic esters to delete viable bacteria by flow cytometry. *J. Appl. Bacteriol.* **77**: 221–228.

Fiering, S.N., Roederer, M., Nolan, G.P., Micklem, D.R., Parks, D.R. and Herzenberg, L.A. (1991) Improved FACS-Gal-flow cytometric analysis and sorting of viable eukaryotic cells expressing reporter gene constructs. *Cytometry* **12**: 291–301.

Gross, H.-J., Verwer, B., Houck, D., Hoffman, R.A. and Recktenwald, D. (1995) Model study detecting breast cancer cells in peripheral blood mononuclear cells at frequencies as low as 10^{-7}. *Proc. Natl Acad. Sci. USA* **92**: 537–541.

Hoang, T., Gilmore, D., Metcalf, D., Cobbold, S., Watt, S., Clark, M., Furth, M. and Waldmann, H. (1983) Separation of hemopoietic cells from adult mouse marrow by use of monoclonal antibodies. *Blood* **61**: 580–588.

Jepras, R.I., Carter, J., Pearson, S.C., Paul, F.E. and Wilkinson, M.J. (1995) Development of a robust flow cytometric assay for determining numbers of viable bacteria. *Appl. Environ. Microbiol.* **61**: 2696–2701.

Kaprelyants, A.S. and Kell, D.B. (1992) Rapid assessment of bacterial viability and vitality by rhodamine 123 and flow cytometry. *J. Appl. Bacteriol.* **72**: 410–422.

Loken, M.R. and Lanier, L.L. (1984) Three-color immunofluorescence analysis of Leu antigens on human peripheral blood using two lasers on a fluorescence activated cell sorter. *Cytometry* **5**: 151–158.

Nicola, N.A., Metcalf, D., von Melchner, H. and Burgess, A.W. (1981) Isolation of murine fetal hemopoietic progenitor cells and selective fractionation of various erythroid precursors. *Blood* **58**: 376–386.

Ormerod, M.G. (ed.) (1994) *Flow Cytometry: A Practical Approach,* 2nd Edn. IRL Press at Oxford University Press, Oxford.

Sartor, M. and Bradstock, K. (1994) Detection of intracellular lymphoid differentiation antigens by flow cytometry in acute lymphoblastic leukemia. *Cytometry* **18**: 119–122.

Protocol 6.1

Checklist for initial steps in setting up a flow sorter

Protocol

1. Ensure that sheath fluid or liquid reservoir contains buffered saline solution.

2. Switch on the instrument and set-up as for normal analysis.

3. Check that stream is central between deflection plates. To ensure stable flow conditions, leave stream to run for 30 min.

4. Select correct transducer frequency for flow chamber orifice diameter.

5. Switch on transducer. Adjust transducer amplitude to minimize the break-off distance and number of satellite droplets.

6. Switch on high voltage on deflection plates and test charging pulse.

7. Adjust phase of the charging pulse to give two sharp side streams.

8. Adjust charge pulse amplitude to give desired amount of deflection.

9. Switch off test pulse and set droplet delay time as instructed in manufacturer's manual.

Notes

Preliminary analysis of sample to be sorted may be performed whilst ensuring stable flow conditions.

Droplet formation can be observed using a 'built-in' small strobed light source.

Failure to obtain sharp side streams is usually caused by dirt in the flow chamber orifice.

Protocol 6.2

Guide to checking droplet delay time

Procedure

1. After initial set-up of cytometer, run a test sample in the cytometer.

2. Select a gate to sort cells (or fluorescent beads) to the left.

3. Select one droplet sorting; decrease droplet delay time by two.

4. Sort a given number of cells (or beads) (50–100) on to a microscope slide.

5. Increase drop delay time by one unit, move microscope slide to a fresh area, and repeat sort.

6. Repeat a further three times.

7. Using a microscope, count the number of cells (or beads) in each drop. If the cells (or beads) are shared between two droplets adjust drop delay time. The aim is to have 90% or more of the cells in a single drop.

8. If necessary, adjust drop delay time to that of the drop that contained the sorted cells.

Notes

Test sample can be either the sample to be sorted or some fluorescent beads.

Drops will be nicely formed if the slide is slightly greasy. This is achieved by running ones thumb over the surface of the microscope slide before using it.

When adjusting drop delay time in step 7, if drop delay can be set in fractions of a transducer wavelength, make a small, fractional, change to drop delay time and repeat step 4, etc.

When adjusting drop delay time in step 7, if drop delay can only be set in integers of the drop period, switch off the sample flow, switch on the test pulse, make small change to transducer amplitude, adjust phase of the charging pulse to obtain sharp side streams, turn off test pulse, re-run sample, and repeat step 4, etc.

Several types of beads are available including FluoroSpheres (DAKO) and Quantum Simply Cellular Beads (Sigma).

Protocol 6.3

Checklist for measuring the yield of sorted cells

Protocol

1. Before sorting, measure the concentration of cells in the sample.

2. Weigh the sample and collection tubes.

3. During initial flow cytometric analysis, record percentage of cells in the gate selected for sorting.

4. Carry out sort and collect fractions.

5. Weigh the sample and collection tubes. The difference in weight before and after sorting will determine the volume of cells that passed through the sorter and the volume of cells collected.

6. Calculate the number of selected cells that passed through the sorter (i.e. sample volume × concentration × percentage of cells gated).

7. Measure the concentration of cells in the sorted sample.

8. Reanalyze an aliquot of the sorted cells to measure purity.

9. Calculate the number of sorted cells (i.e. collected volume × concentration × purity).

10. Calculate percentage yield (i.e. number of sorted cells ÷ number of selected cells × 100).

Protocol 6.4

Precautions taken to maintain sterility

Procedure

Sheath tubing

1. Pass sterilizing fluid, such as 1% hypochlorite, through the sheath fluid assembly.

2. Wash through with sterile, filtered (0.2 μm) water for at least 15 min.

3. Wash through with sterile sheath fluid.

Sample collection

1. Clean all surfaces around the sample collection point.

2. Wipe down with disinfectant such as 70% ethanol.

3. Enclose the area during the sort.

Sample delivery

1. Pass dilute bleach through the sample delivery system.

2. Flush through with sterile, filtered (0.2 μm) water for at least 15 min. It is wise to do this after the instrument has been adjusted for correct sorting and immediately before running the sample.

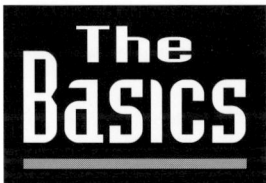

List of manufacturers and suppliers

Many of the larger companies have subsidiaries in other countries while most of the smaller companies market their products themselves or through agents. The name of a local supplier can be obtained by contacting the relevant company listed here. The numbers bracketed are area, freephone or freefax code numbers; international dialing codes have not been listed. UK (0800) and USA (800) freephone or freefax numbers can only be used in the corresponding countries.

Accurate Chemical & Scientific Corporation, 300 Shames Drive, Westbury, NY 11590, USA.

Advanced Magnetics Inc., 61 Mooney Street, Cambridge, Massachusetts 02138-1038, USA.

Amersham Pharmacia Biotech Ltd., Amersham Place, Little Chalfont, Bucks HP7 9NA, UK. Tel. (0870) 606 1921. Fax. (01494) 544350.
Amersham Pharmacia Biotech Inc., 800 Centennial Avenue, PO Box 1327, Piscataway, NJ 08855-1327, USA. Tel. (732) 457 8000. Fax. (732) 457 0557.

Anachem Ltd., 20 Charles Street, Luton, Beds., LU2 0EB, UK. Tel. (01582) 745000. Fax. (01582) 488815.

Anderman and Co. Ltd., 145 London Road, Kingston-Upon-Thames, Surrey KT17 7NH, UK.

Beckman Coulter, Oakley Court, Kingsmead Business Park, London Road, High Wycombe, Bucks HP11 1JU, UK. Tel. (01494) 441181. Fax. (01494) 447558.
Beckman Instruments Inc., 2500 Harbor Boulevard, Box 3100, Fullerton, CA 92634-3100, USA. Tel. (800) 742 2345. Fax. (800) 643 4366.

Becton Dickinson UK Ltd, Between Towns Road, Cowley, Oxford OX4 3LY, UK. Tel. (01865) 748844. Fax. (01865) 781635.
Becton Dickinson, 2350 Qume Drive, San Jose, CA 95131-1807, USA. Tel. (800) 223 8226.

Bibby Sterilin, Tilling Drive, Stone, Staffs ST15 0SA, UK. Tel. (01785) 812121. Fax. (01785) 813748.
Bibby Sterilin (Dynalon), PO Box 112, Rochester, NY 146001-0112, USA. Tel. (716) 334 2060. Fax. (716) 334 9496.

Bio-Rad Laboratories Ltd., Bio-Rad House, Maylands Avenue, Hemel Hempstead, Herts HP2 7TD, UK. Tel. (020) 8328 2000. Fax. (020) 8328 2550.

Bio-Rad Laboratories, 2000 Alfred Nobel Drive, Hercules, CA 94547, USA. Tel. (510) 741 1000. Fax. (510) 741 5800.

Calbiochem, Boulevard Industrial Park, Padge Road, Beeston, Nottingham NG9 2JR, UK. Tel. (0115) 943 0840. Fax. (0115) 943 0951.

Calbiochem Corp., PO Box 12087, La Jolla, CA 92039-2087, USA. Tel. (800) 854 3417. Fax. (800) 776 0999.

Corning Costar UK, 10 The Valley Centre, Gordon Road, High Wycombe, Bucks HP13 6EQ, UK. Tel. (01494) 471207. Fax. (01494) 464891.

Dako Ltd., Denmark House, Angel Drove, Ely, Cambs CB7 4ET, UK. Tel. (01353) 669911. Fax. (01353) 668989.

Dako Corp., 6392 Via Real, Carpinteria, CA 93013, USA. Tel. (805) 566 6655. Fax. (805) 566 6688.

Denley Instruments Ltd., see ThermoQuest

Du Pont (UK) Ltd., see NEN Life Science

Dynal Ltd. UK, 11 Bassendale Road, Croft Business Park, Bromborough, Wirral CH62 3QL, UK. Tel. (0151) 346 1234. Fax. (0151) 346 1223.

Dynal Inc, 5 Delaware Drive., Lake Success, NY 11042, USA. Tel. (516) 326 3270. Fax. (516) 326 3298.

Fisher Scientific UK, Bishop Meadow Road, Loughborough, Leics LE11 5RG, UK. Tel. (01509) 231166. Fax. (01509) 231893.

Heraeus Equipment Ltd., 9 Wates Way, Brentwood, Essex CM15 9TD, UK. Tel. (01277) 231511. Fax. (01277) 261856.

Hitachi Scientific Instruments, Hogwood Industrial Estate, Finchhampstead, UK. Tel. (01734) 328632. Fax. (01734) 328779.

ICN Biomedical Ltd., 1 Elmwood, Chineham Business Park, Basingstoke, Hamps RG24 8WG, UK. Tel. (0800) 282474. Fax. (0800) 614735.

ICN Biomedical Inc., 3300 Hyland Av., Costa Mesa, CA 92626, USA. Tel. (714) 545 0100. Fax. (714) 557 4872.

Life Technologies Ltd., 3 Fountain Drive, Inchinnan Business Park, Paisley PA4 9RF, UK Tel. (0141) 814 6100. Fax. (0141) 814 6287.

Medipharm, see Nycomed Amersham.

Merck Ltd., Hunter Boulevard, Magna Park, Lutterworth, Leics LE17 4XN, UK. Tel. (0800) 223344. Fax. (01455) 558586.

Miltenyi Biotec Ltd., Almac House, Church Lane, Bisley, Surrey GU24 9DR, UK. Tel. (01483) 799800. Fax. (01438) 799811.

Miltenyi Biotec Inc., 251 Auburn Ravine Road, Suite 208, Auburn, CA 95603, USA. Tel. (530) 888 8871. Fax. (530) 888 8925.

Molecular Dynamics Ltd., 5 Beech House, Chiltern Court. Tel. (01494) 793377. Fax. (01494) 793222

Nalge Nunc International, Foxwood Court, Rotherwas, Hereford HR2 6JQ, UK. Tel. (01432) 263933. Fax. (01432) 351923.

Nalge Nunc International, PO Box 20365, Rochester, NY 14602-0365, USA. Tel. (716) 264 3898. Fax. (716) 264 3706.

NEN Life Science Products, BRU/BRU/40349, PO Box 66, Hounslow TW5 9RT, UK. Tel. (0800) 896046. Fax. (0800) 891714.

NEN Life Science Products Inc., 549-3 Albany Street, Boston, MA 02118, USA. Tel. (617) 482 9595. Fax. (617) 482 1380.

New England Biolabs Ltd., 73 Knowl Piece, Wilbury Way, Hitchin, Herts SG4 0TY, UK. Tel. (01462) 420616. Fax. (01462) 421057.

New England Biolabs Inc., 32 Tozer Road, Beverly, MA 01915-5599, USA. Tel. (978) 927 5054. Fax. (978) 921 1350.

Nycomed Amersham, see Amersham Pharmacia Biotech UK.

Philip Harris Scientific, Novara House, Excelsior Road, Ashby Park, Ashby de la Zouch, Leics LE65 1NG, UK. Tel. (0845) 604090. Fax. (01530) 419300.

Promega UK Ltd., Delta House, Chilworth Research Centre, Southampton SO16 7NS, UK. Tel. (023) 8076 0225. Fax. (023) 8076 7014.

Promega Corp., 2800 Woods Hollow Road, Madison, WI 53711-5399, USA. Tel. (608) 274 4330. Fax. (608) 277 2516.

R & D Systems Ltd., 4-10 The Quadrant, Barton Lane, Abingdon, Oxon OX14 3YS, UK. Tel. (01235) 551100. Fax. (01235) 533420.

R & D Systems Inc., 614 McKinley Place, Minneapolis, MN 55413 USA. Tel. (800) 343 7475. Fax. (612) 379 6580.

Roche Diagnostics Ltd., Bell Lane, Lewes, East Sussex BN7 1LG, UK. Tel. (01273) 480444. Fax. (01273) 480266.

Roche Diagnostics Corp., 9115 Hague Road, PO Box 50414, Indianapolis, IN 46250-0414, USA. Tel. (800) 428 5433. Fax. (800) 428 2883.

Sanyo Gallenkamp Plc., Park House, Meridian East, Meridian Business Park, Leicester LE3 2UZ, UK. Tel. (0116) 2630530. Fax. (0116) 2620353.

Sarstedt Ltd., 68 Boston Td., Beaumont Leys, Leicester LE4 1AW, UK. Tel. (0116) 2359023. Fax. (0116) 2366099.

Sigma-Aldrich Company Ltd., Fancy Road, Poole, Dorset BH12 4QH, UK. Tel. (01202) 733114. Fax. (0800) 378785.

Sigma Chemical Co., 3050 Spruce Street, St. Louis, MO 63178, USA. Tel. (800) 325 3010. Fax. (800) 325 5052.

ThermoQuest Scientific Equipment Group Ltd., Unit 5, The Ringway Centre, Edison Road, Basingstoke, Hants RG21 6YH, UK. Tel. (01256) 817282. Fax. (01256) 817292.

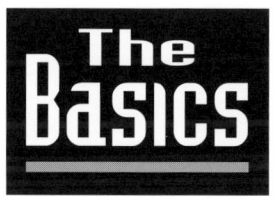

Index